Brave Bear Says Bye-Bye to Tonsils

A Story for Kids About Feeling Brave During Surgery

ISBN: 978-1-7352857-4-0

Written by Stacie C. Skiano, M.S., PA-C

Illustrated by Ralph Skiano

First edition

Brave Little Patients™ is a pediatric support brand dedicated to helping children and their families prepare for medical experiences with courage, clarity, and compassion.

Disclaimer:

This book is for informational and educational purposes only and is not a substitute for professional medical advice, diagnosis, or treatment. Always seek the advice of your child's physician or other qualified healthcare provider with any questions you may have regarding a medical condition.

For more Brave Bear stories and pediatric support resources, visit:

www.BraveLittlePatients.com

Printed in the United States of America

Cover and interior design by Brave Little Patients™

About the Author

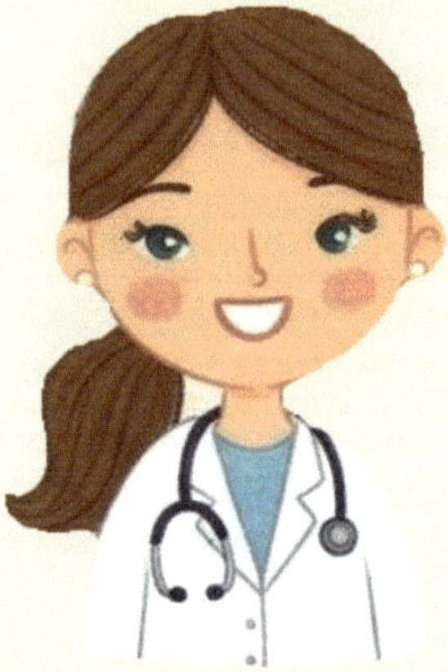

Stacie C. Skiano, M.S., PA-C is a nationally certified Physician Associate and the founder of Brave Little Patients™, a pediatric support platform dedicated to helping families prepare for medical experiences with courage, clarity and compassion. Drawing from years of experience in pediatric surgery and her own journey as a mom, Stacie creates tools to help little ones feel safe, brave, and seen.

To learn more, visit www.bravelittlepatients.com

Medical Review Board

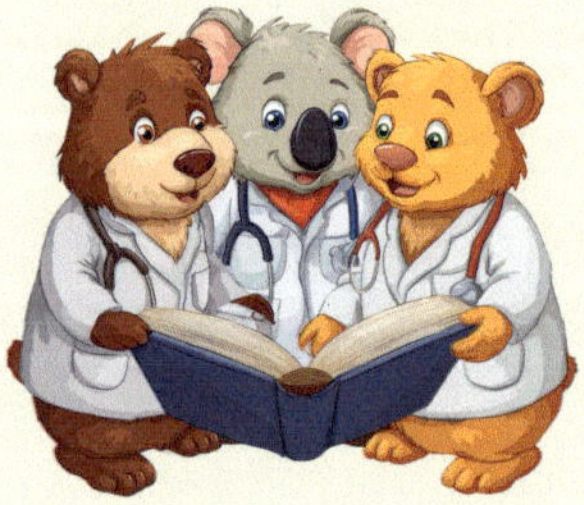

All Brave and Ready stories are reviewed by licensed pediatric medical professionals to ensure accuracy and alignment with evidence-based care practices.

Medical Reviewers for This Title:

Mallory O'Niel, MD - Pediatric Otolaryngology

Bria Bonner, BA, CCLS - Certified Child Life Specialist

Dominik Choromanski, MD - Pediatric Anesthesiology

Tips for reading together:

- Begin talking about the surgery roughly one day per year of your child's age (for example, four days ahead for a four-year-old). Preparing too early can sometimes build worry instead of comfort.
- Read slowly together: Pause often and ask gentle questions like, "Have you ever felt that way too?" This helps your child connect with Brave Bear's story.
- Let your child ask questions—curiosity helps calm fear.
- Practice Brave Bear's breathing techniques together.
- Pack a small bag like Brave Bear to help them feel prepared.

Thank you for making space for emotional preparation. You are your child's biggest support—and Brave Bear is cheering you on, too.

With care,
Stacie

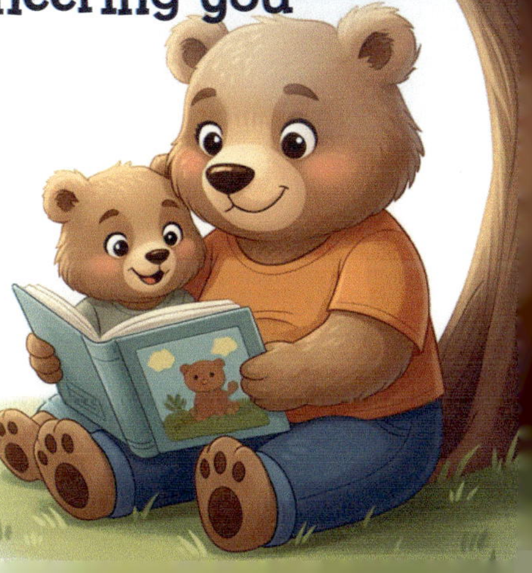

Brave Bear Says Bye-Bye to Tonsils

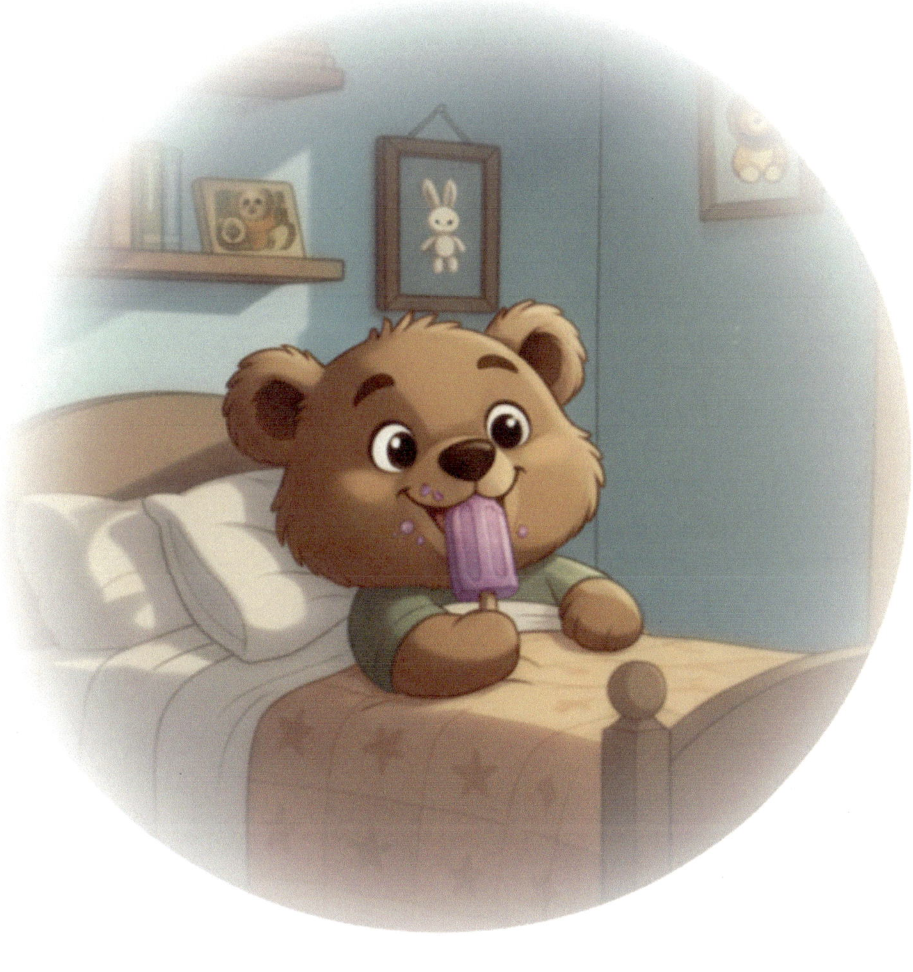

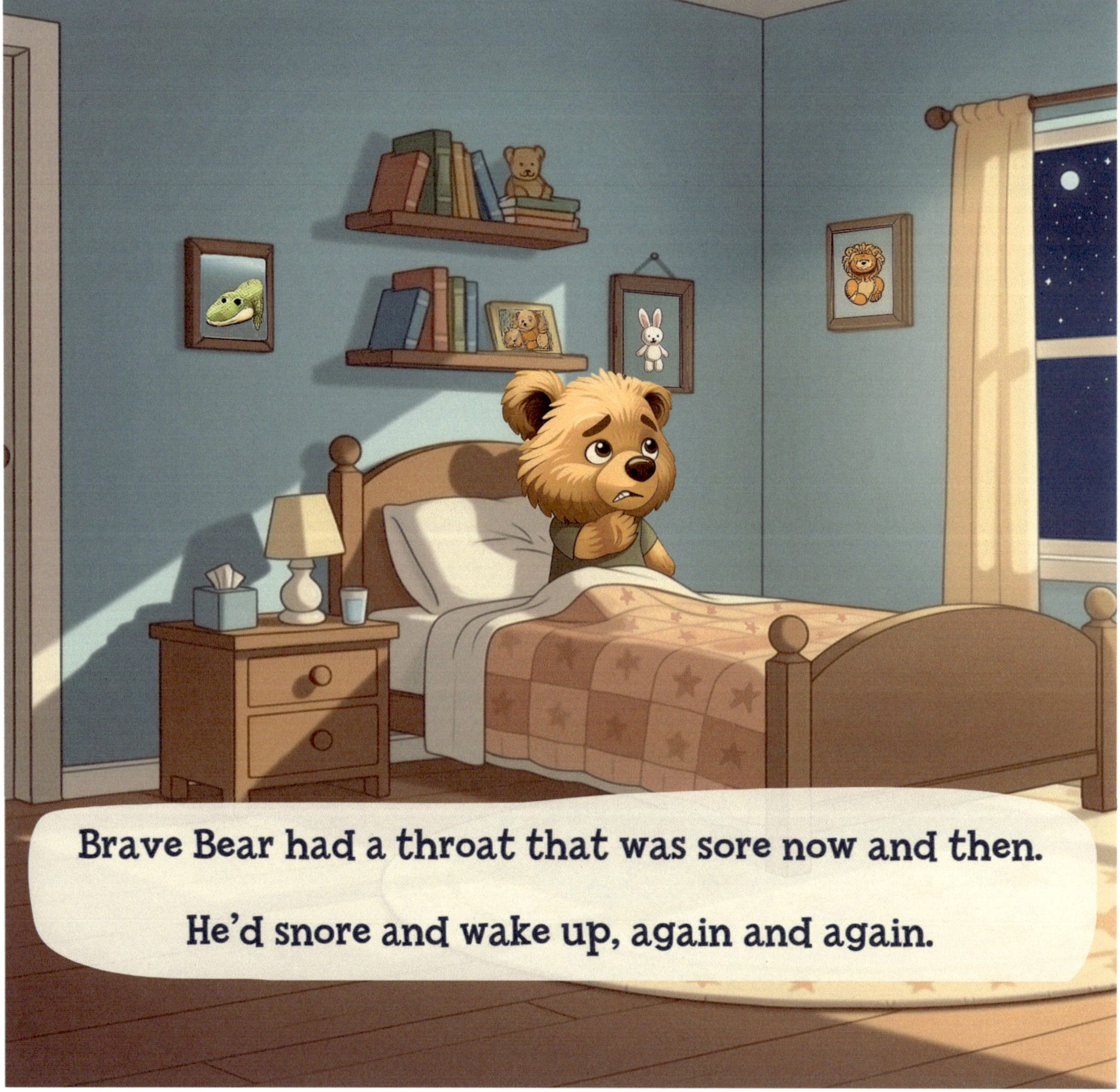

Brave Bear had a throat that was sore now and then.

He'd snore and wake up, again and again.

The nice doctor said, “We can surely help you.”

“We’ll take out your tonsils, you’ll feel good as new!”

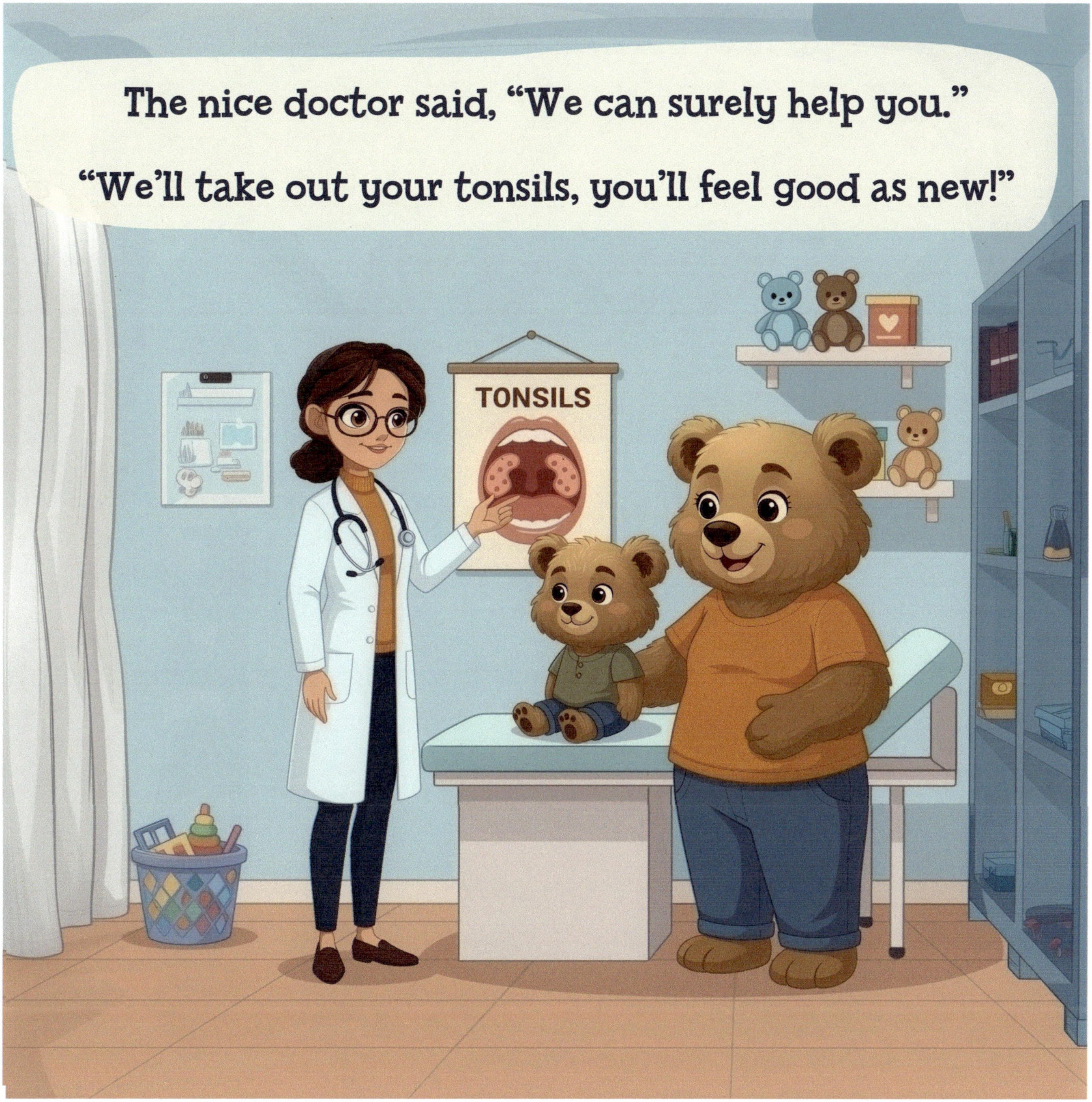

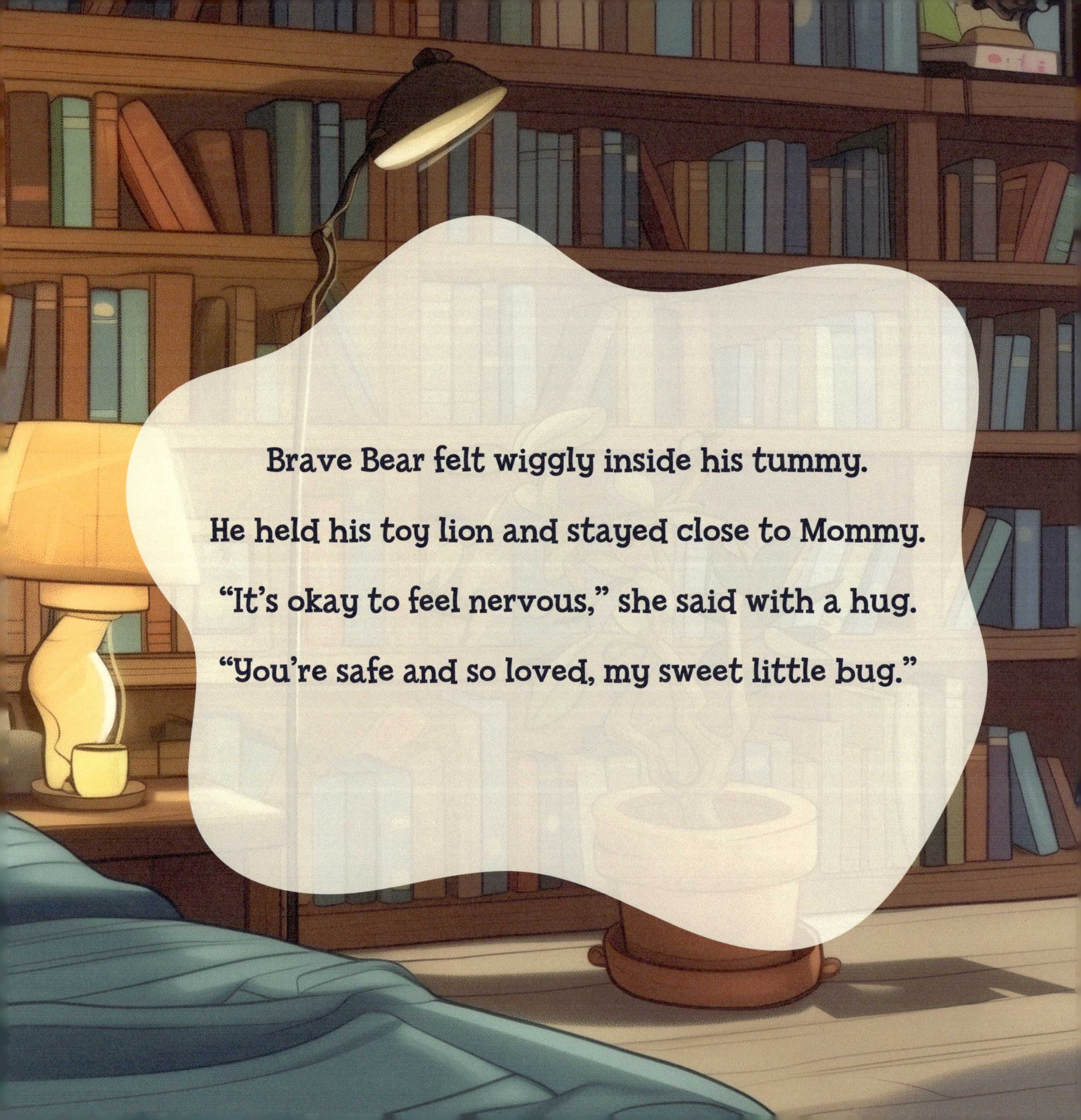

Brave Bear felt wiggly inside his tummy.

He held his toy lion and stayed close to Mommy.

“It’s okay to feel nervous,” she said with a hug.

“You’re safe and so loved, my sweet little bug.”

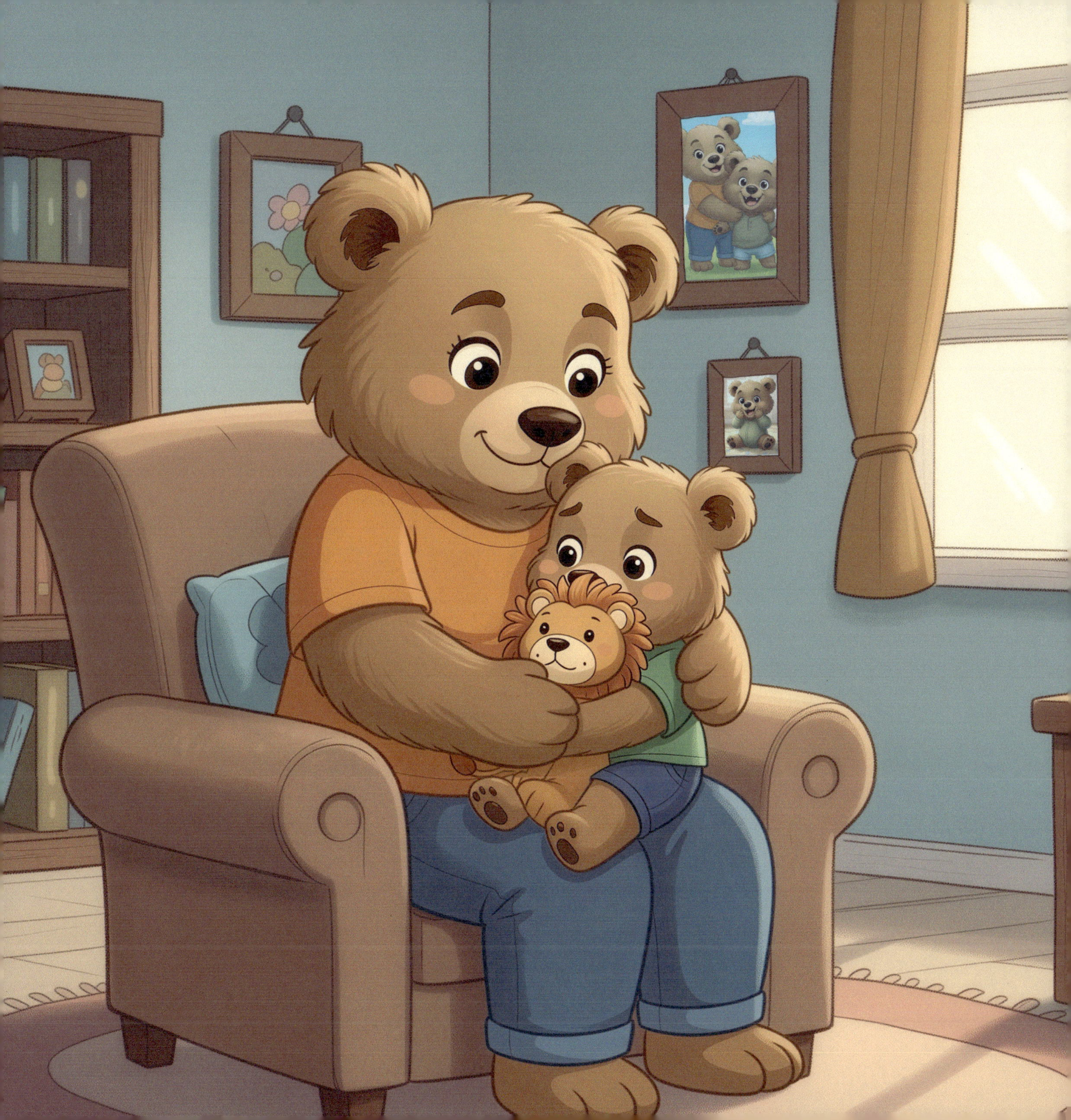

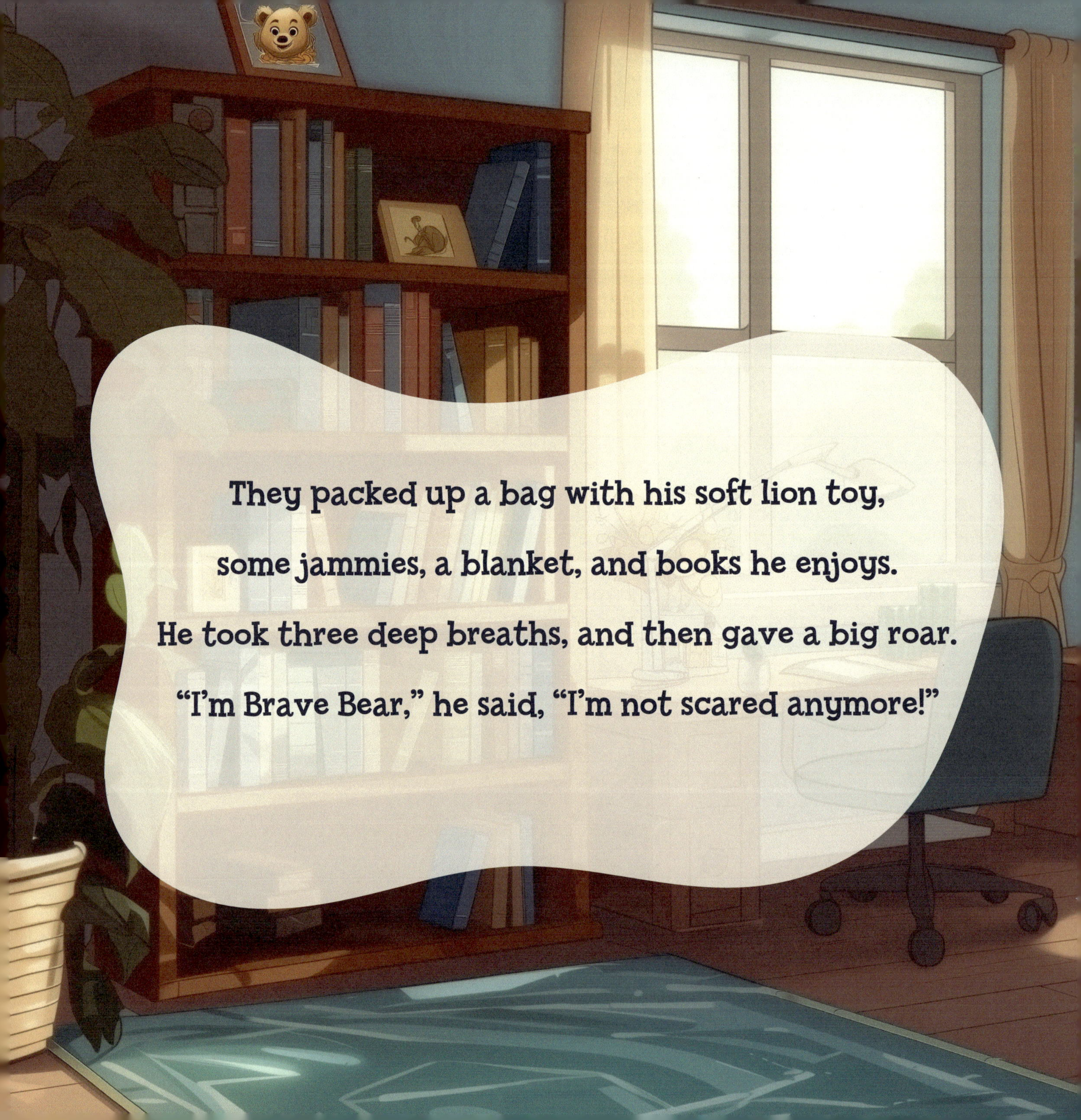

They packed up a bag with his soft lion toy,
some jammies, a blanket, and books he enjoys.
He took three deep breaths, and then gave a big roar.
"I'm Brave Bear," he said, "I'm not scared anymore!"

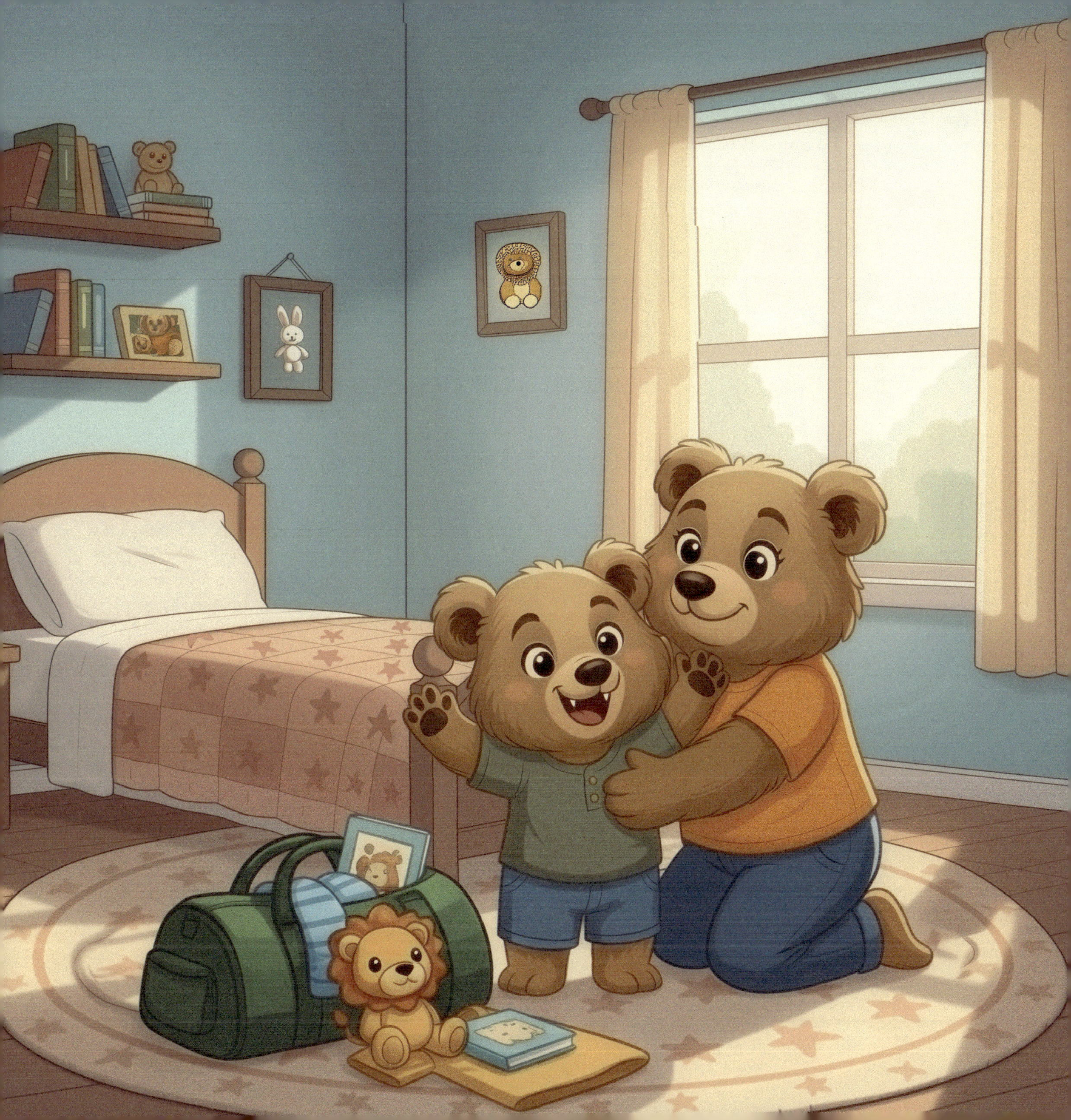

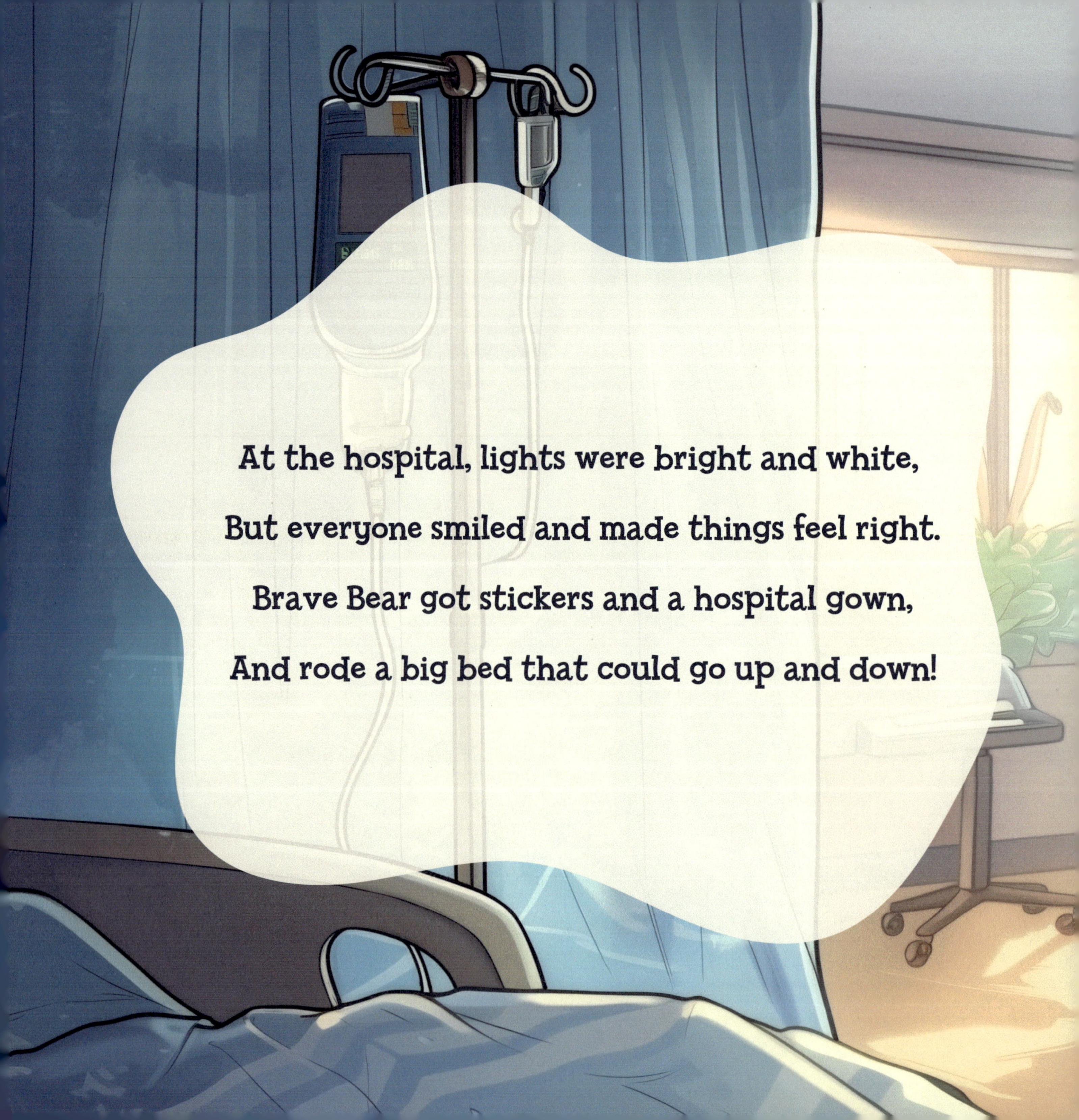

At the hospital, lights were bright and white,

But everyone smiled and made things feel right.

Brave Bear got stickers and a hospital gown,

And rode a big bed that could go up and down!

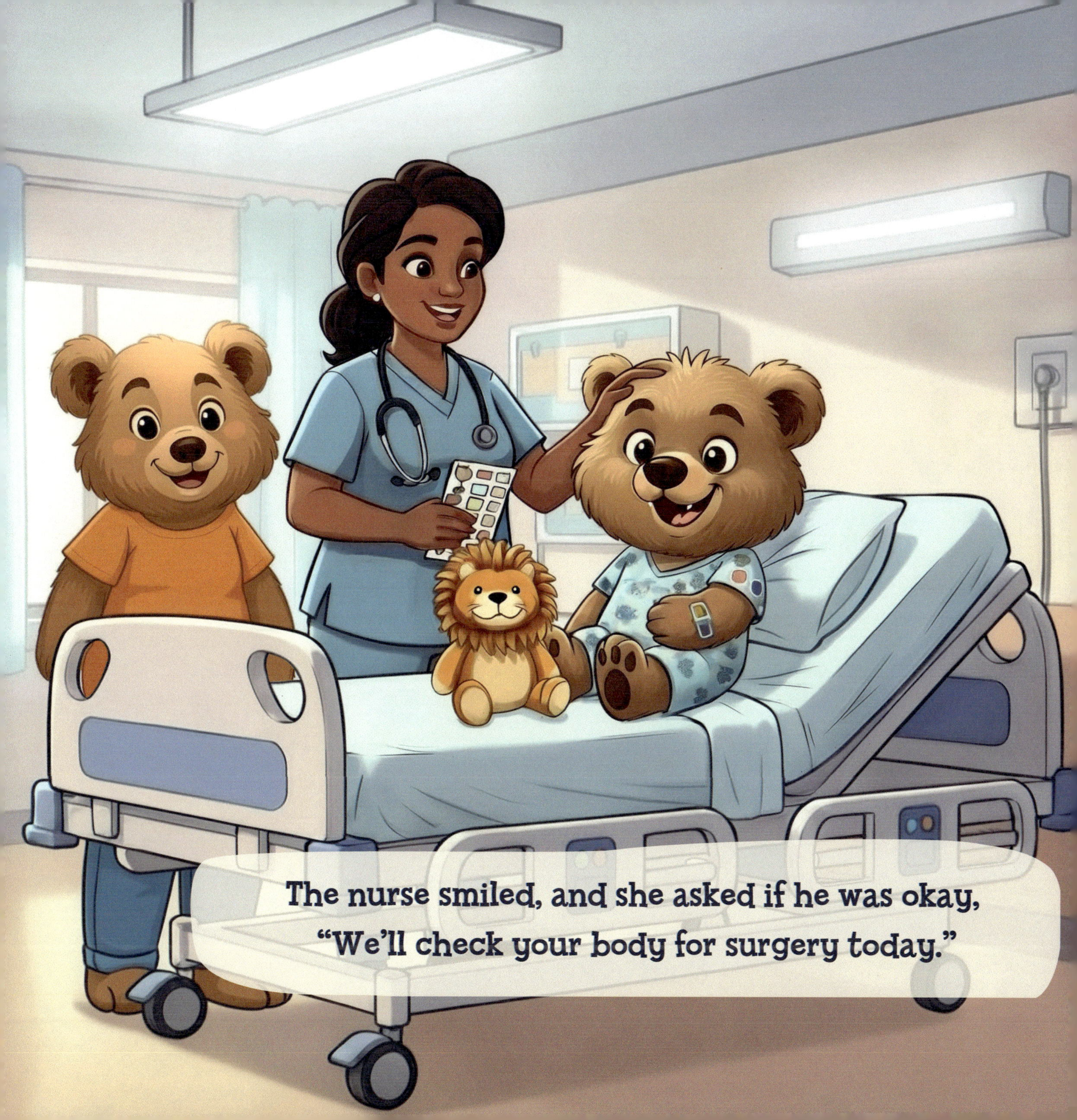

The nurse smiled, and she asked if he was okay,
"We'll check your body for surgery today."

A thermometer swept
across his forehead.
"Your temperature is normal!"
the friendly nurse said.

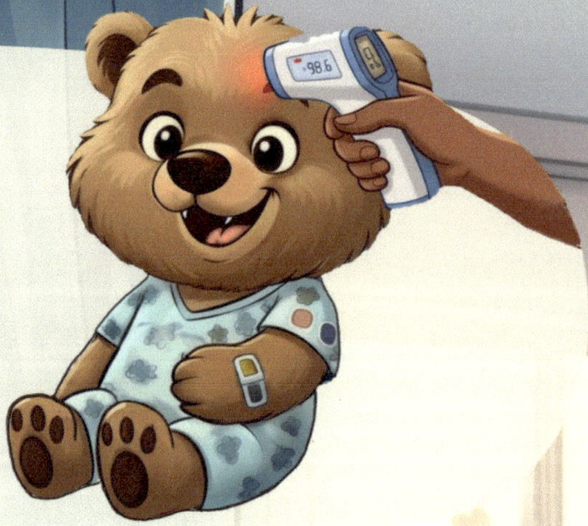

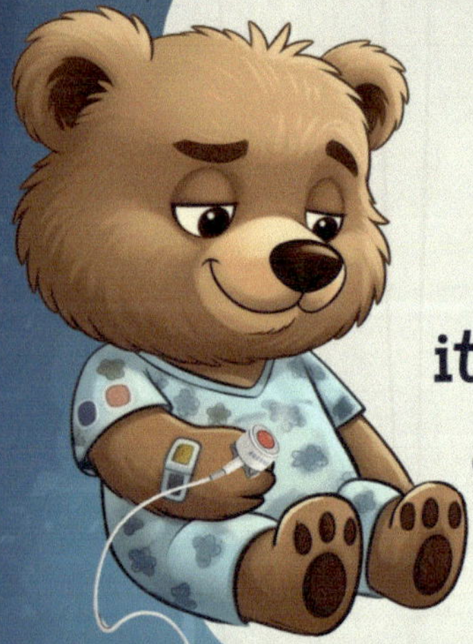

A clip on his finger
shined red on his skin,
it counted his heartbeats,
each breath out and in.

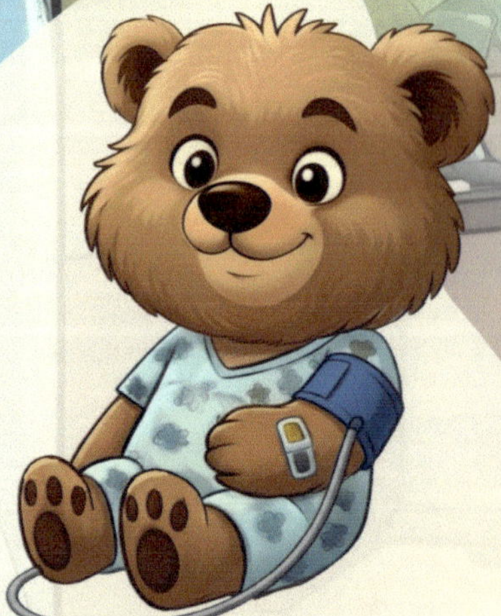

A cuff wrapped his arm,
then gave a big squeeze.
Like a hug it held tight,
then loosened with ease.

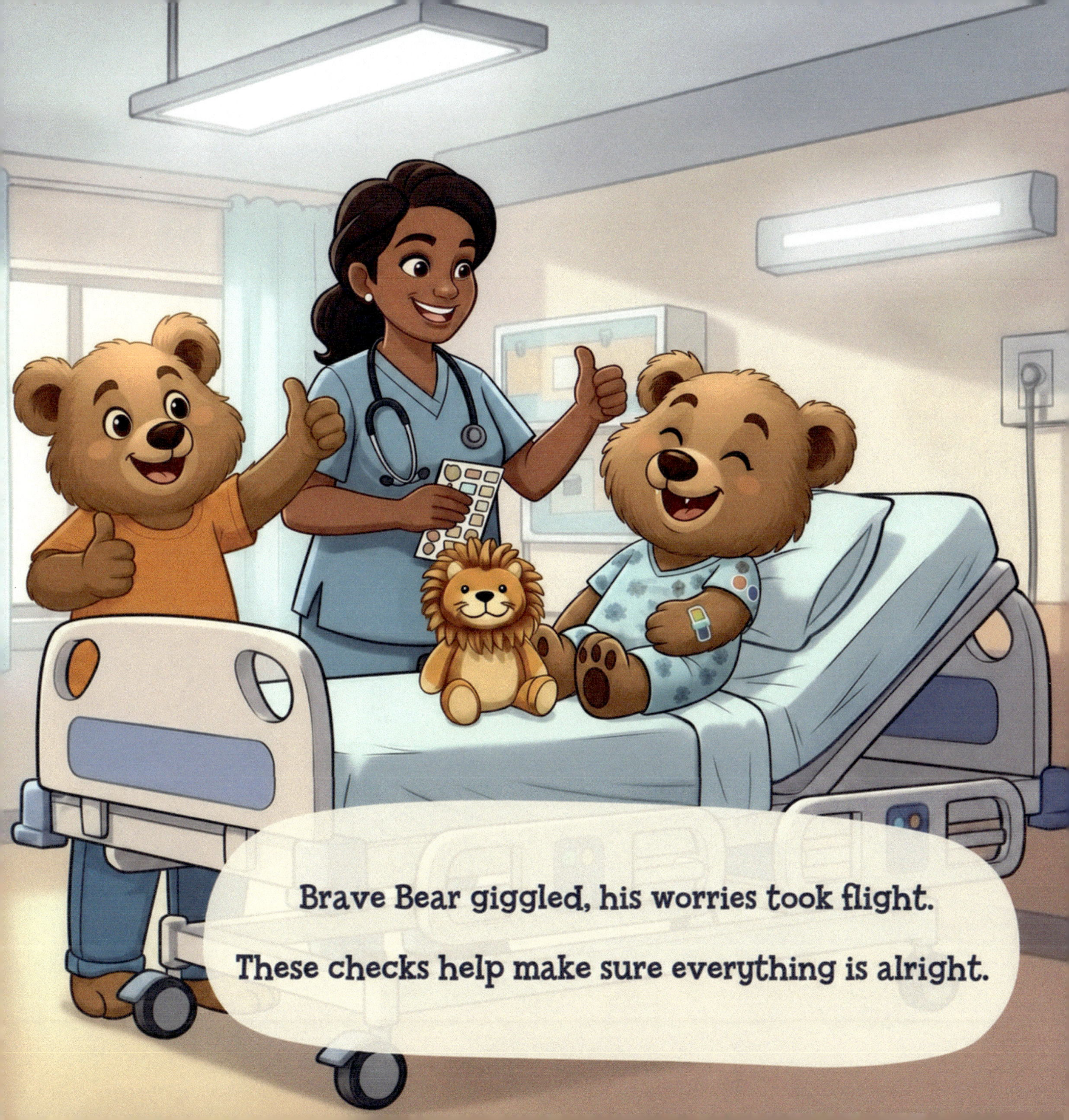

Brave Bear giggled, his worries took flight.

These checks help make sure everything is alright.

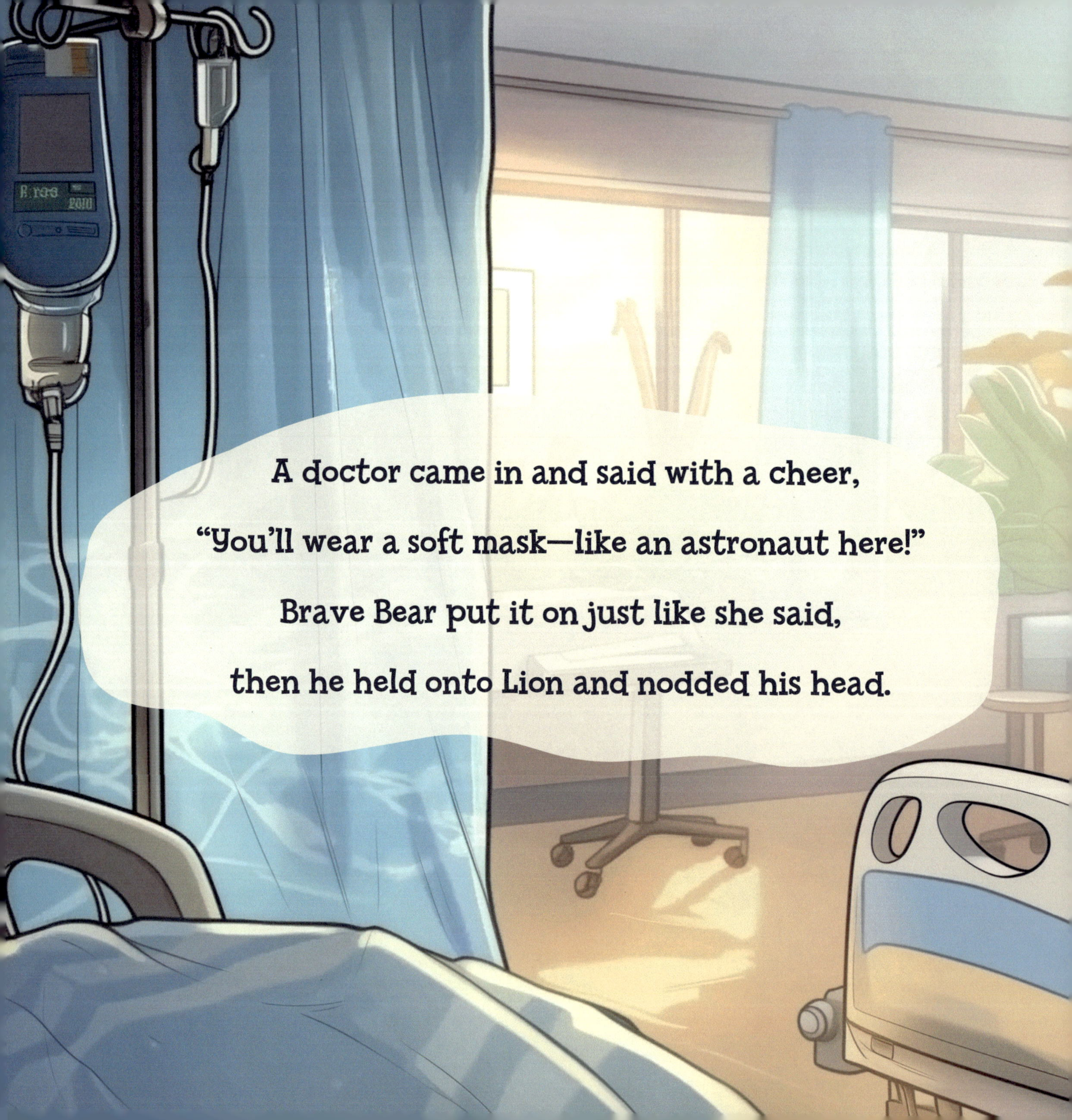

A doctor came in and said with a cheer,

"You'll wear a soft mask—like an astronaut here!"

Brave Bear put it on just like she said,

then he held onto Lion and nodded his head.

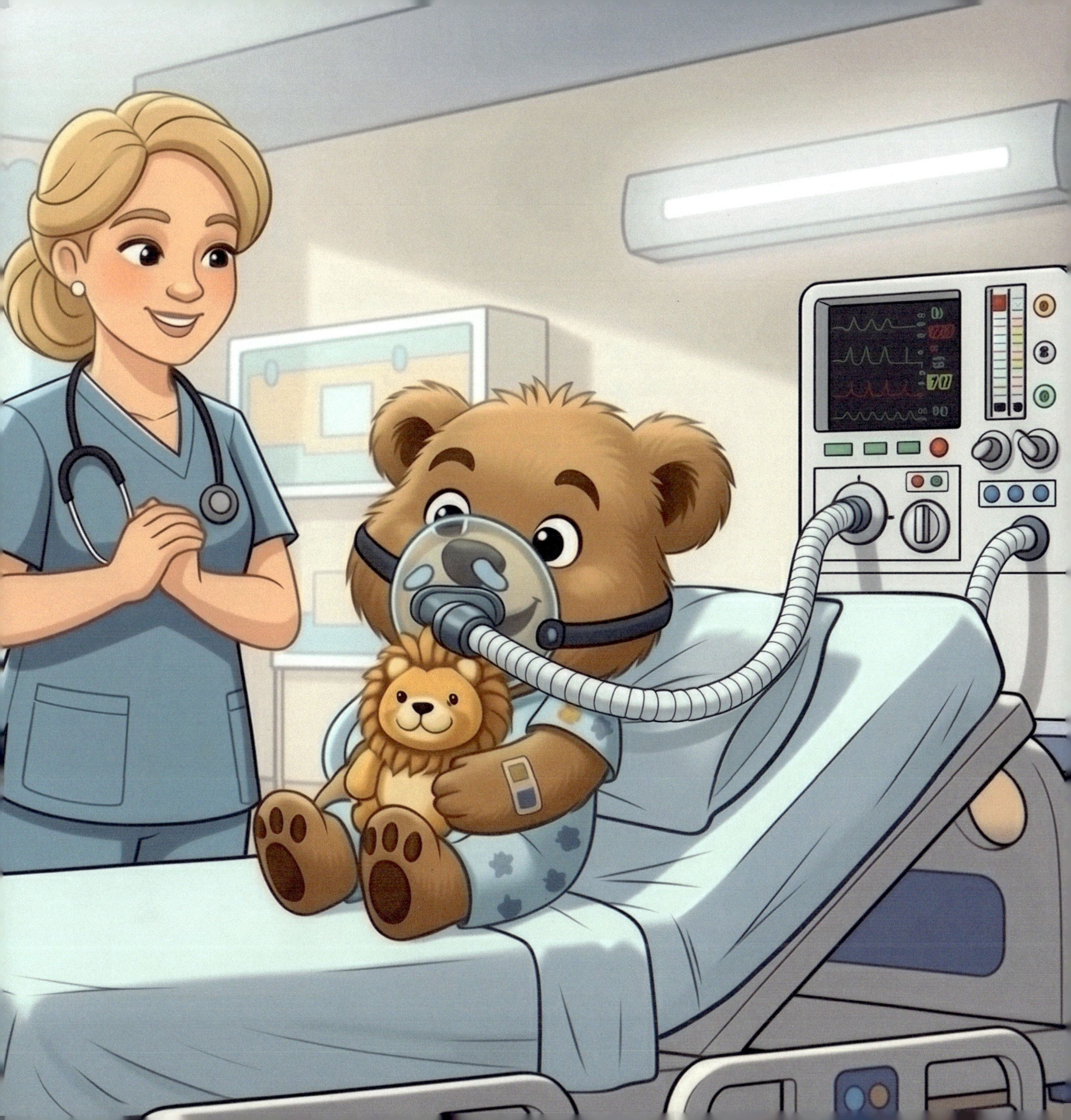

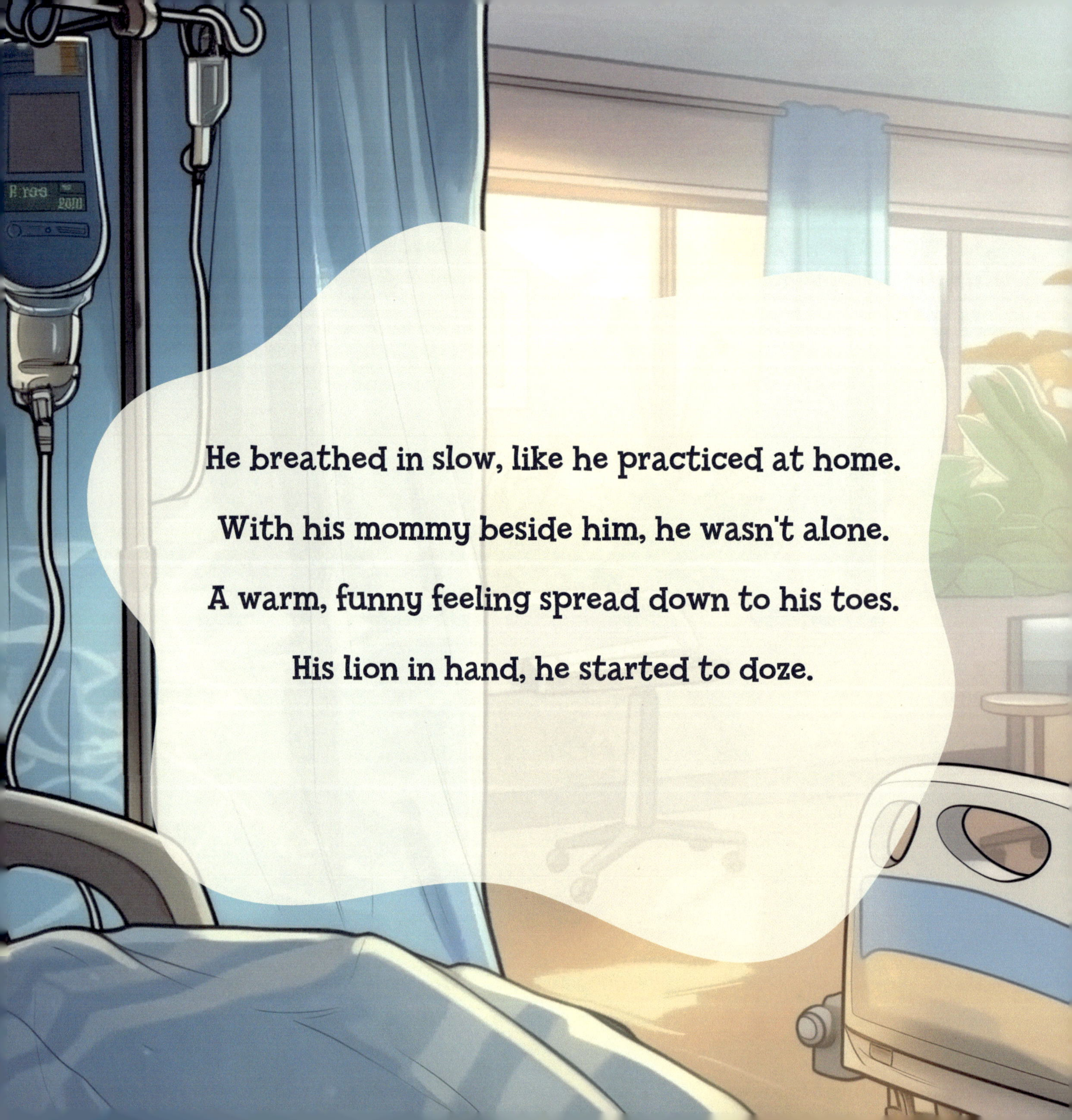

He breathed in slow, like he practiced at home.

With his mommy beside him, he wasn't alone.

A warm, funny feeling spread down to his toes.

His lion in hand, he started to doze.

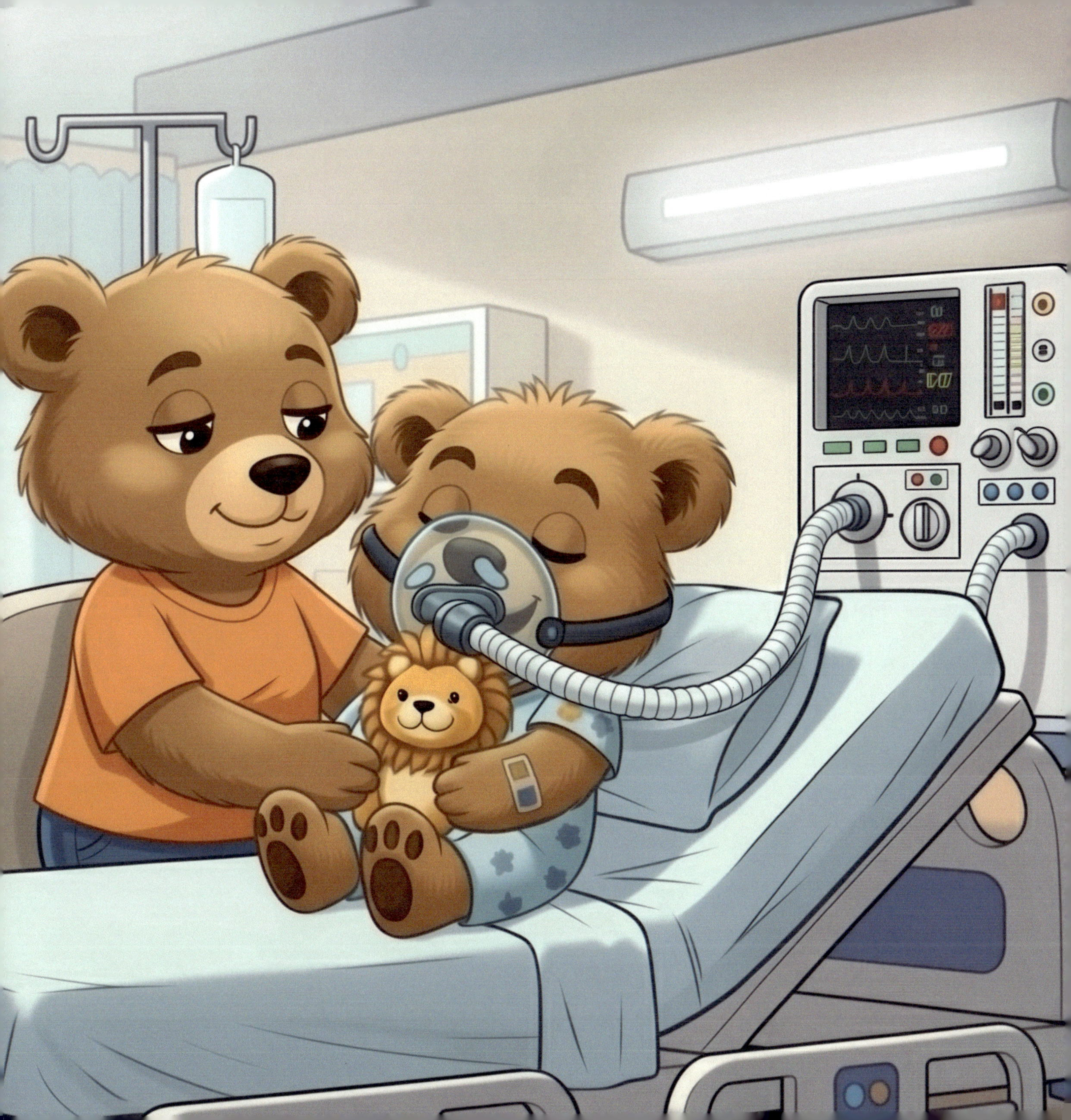

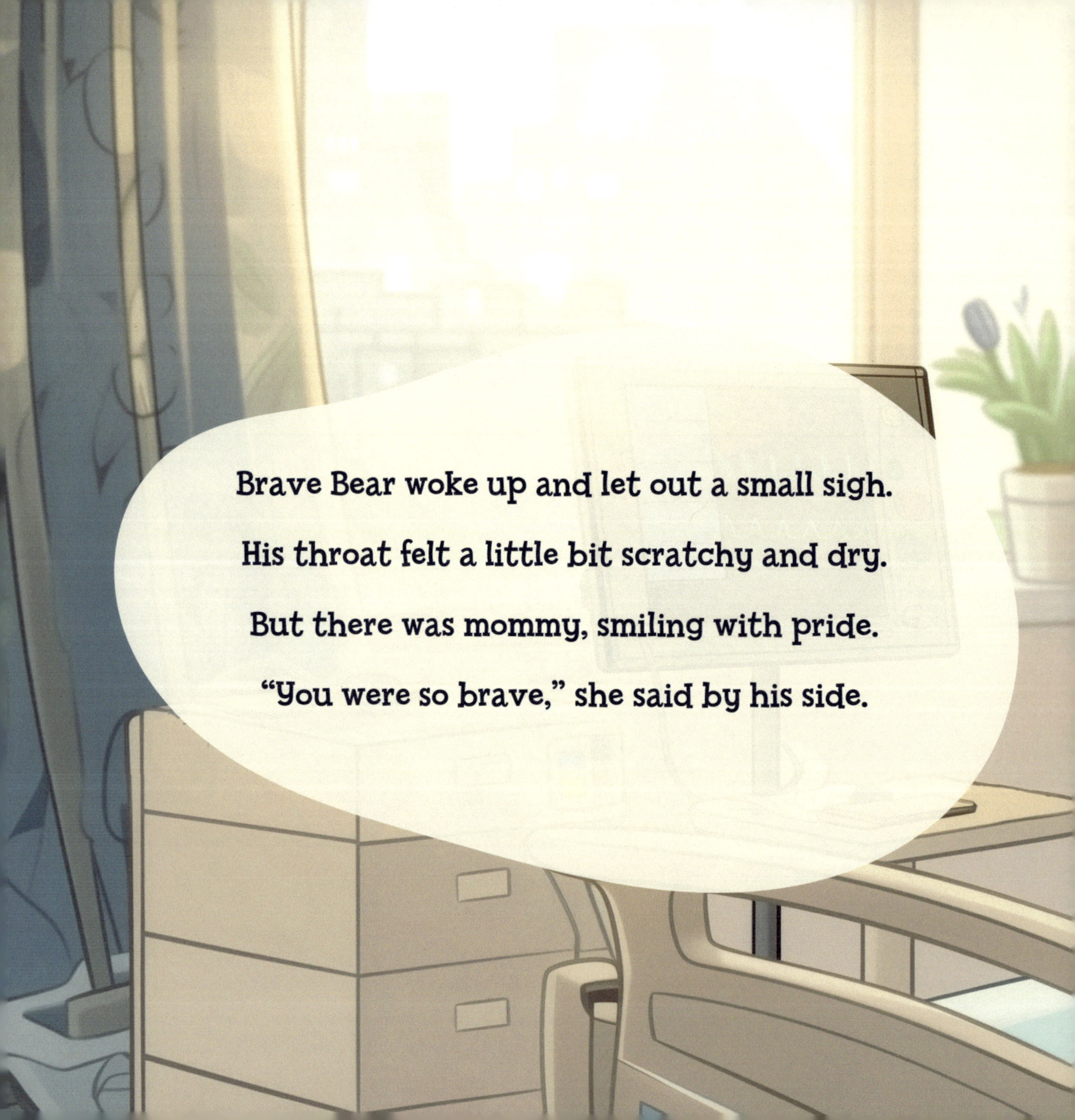

Brave Bear woke up and let out a small sigh.

His throat felt a little bit scratchy and dry.

But there was mommy, smiling with pride.

"You were so brave," she said by his side.

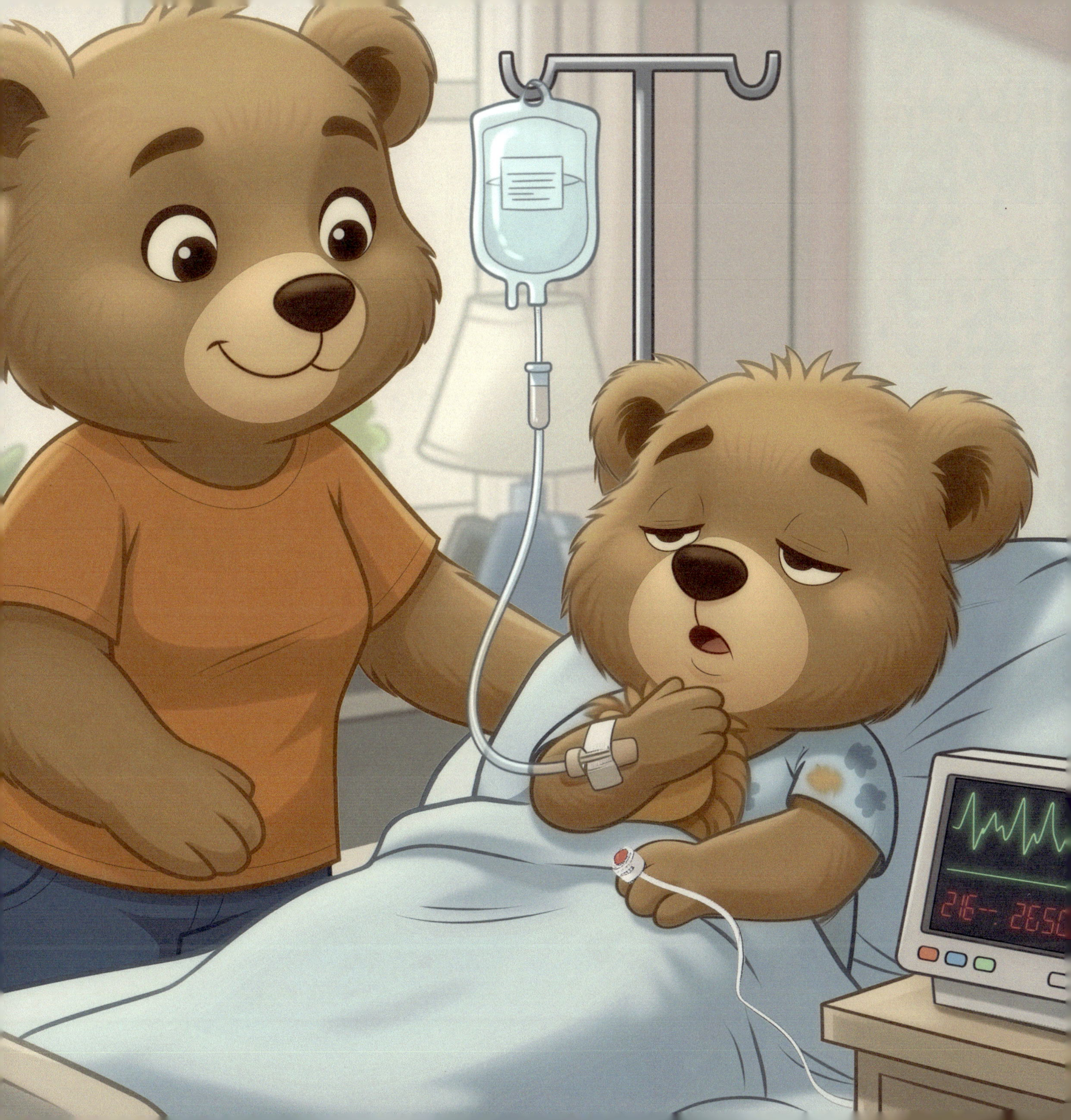

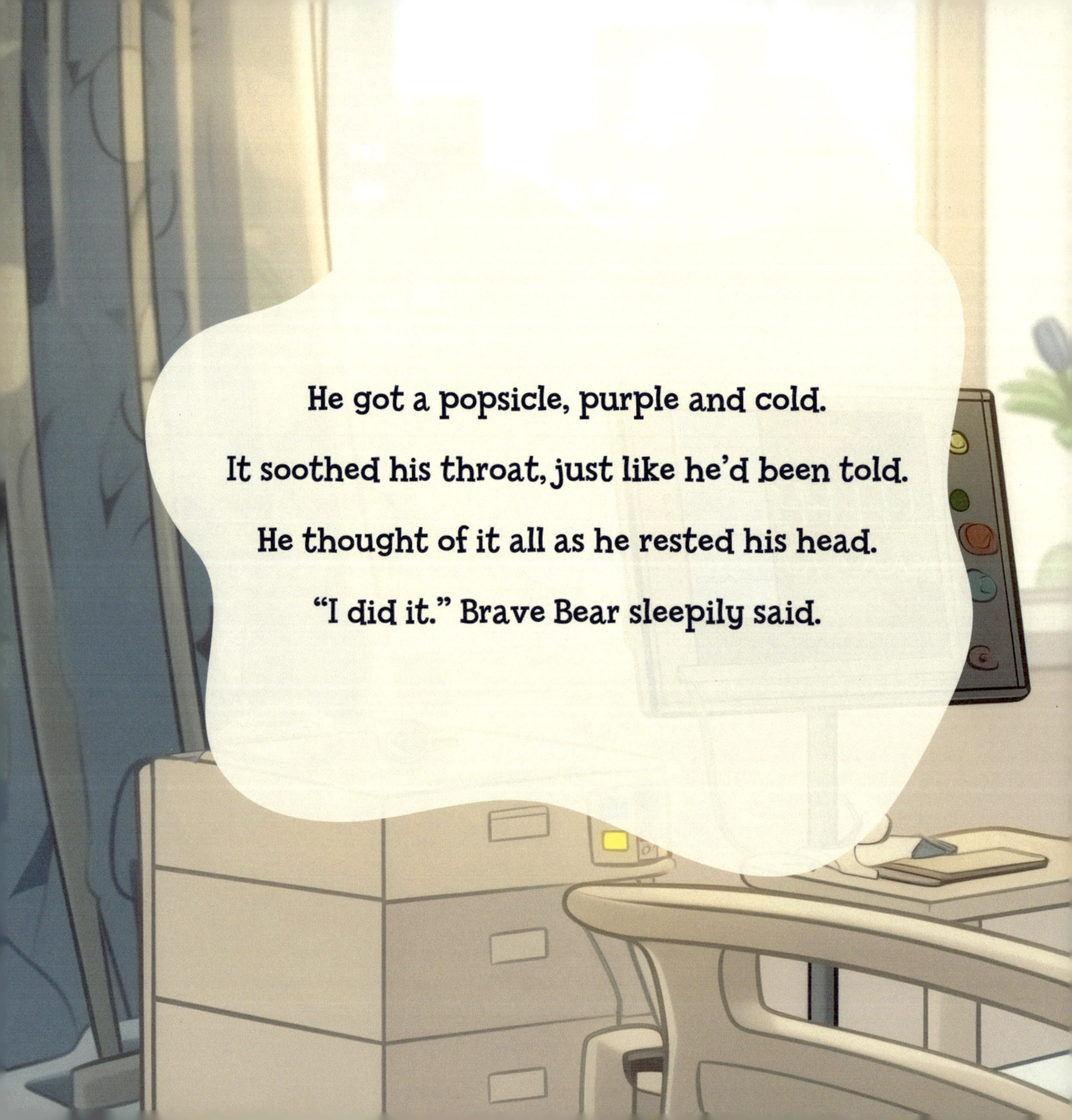

He got a popsicle, purple and cold.

It soothed his throat, just like he'd been told.

He thought of it all as he rested his head.

"I did it." Brave Bear sleepily said.

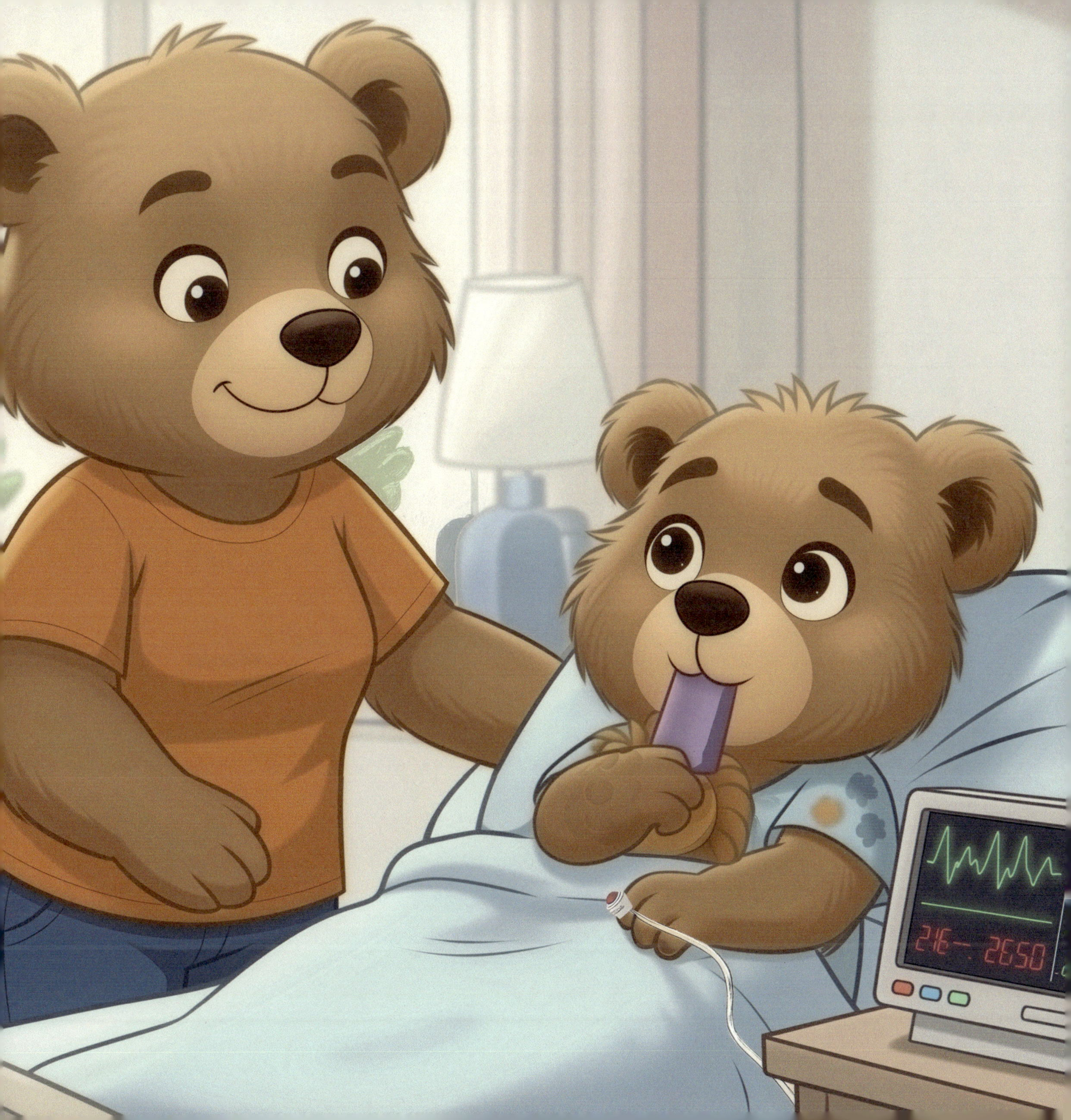

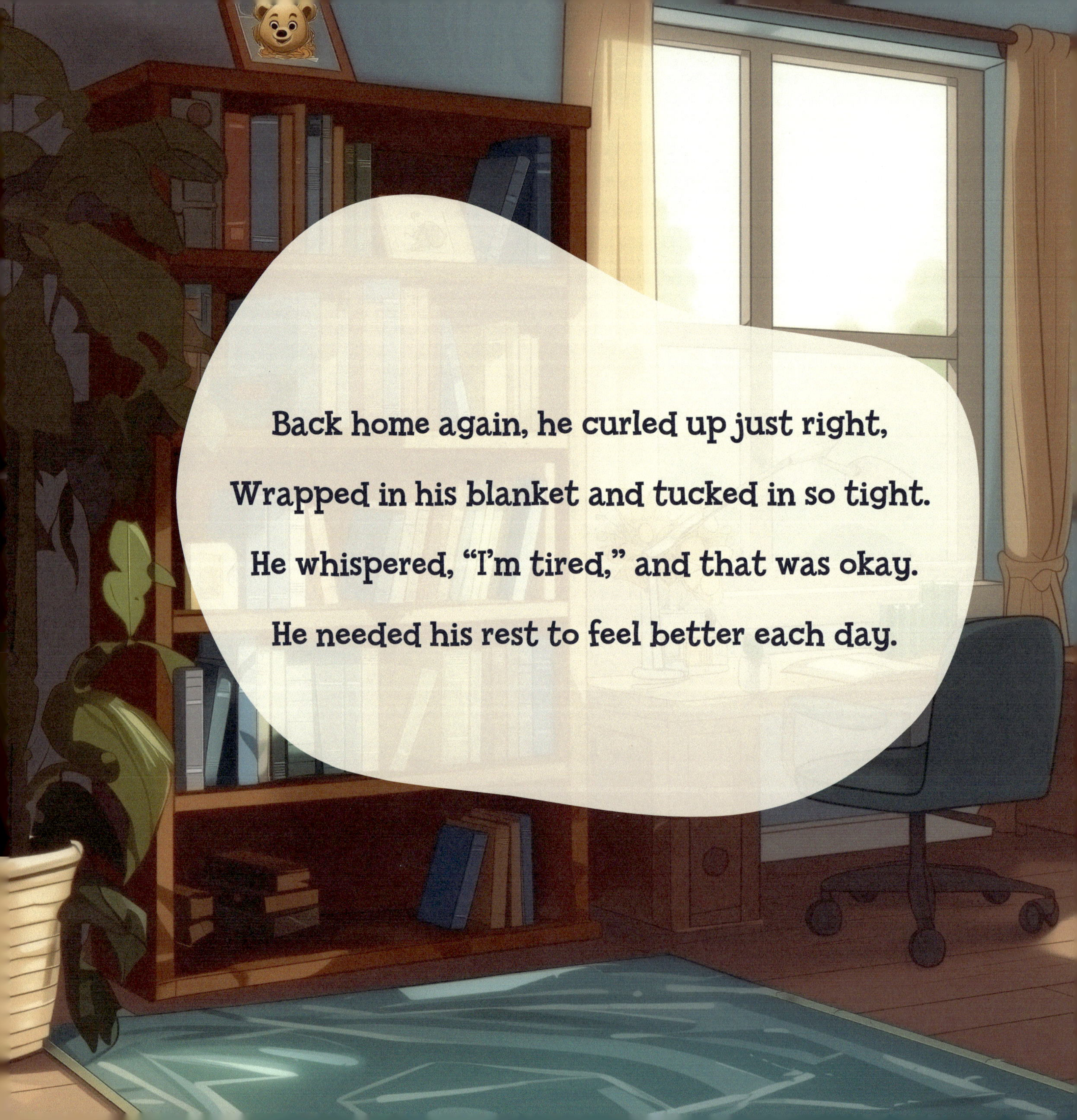

Back home again, he curled up just right,
Wrapped in his blanket and tucked in so tight.
He whispered, "I'm tired," and that was okay.
He needed his rest to feel better each day.

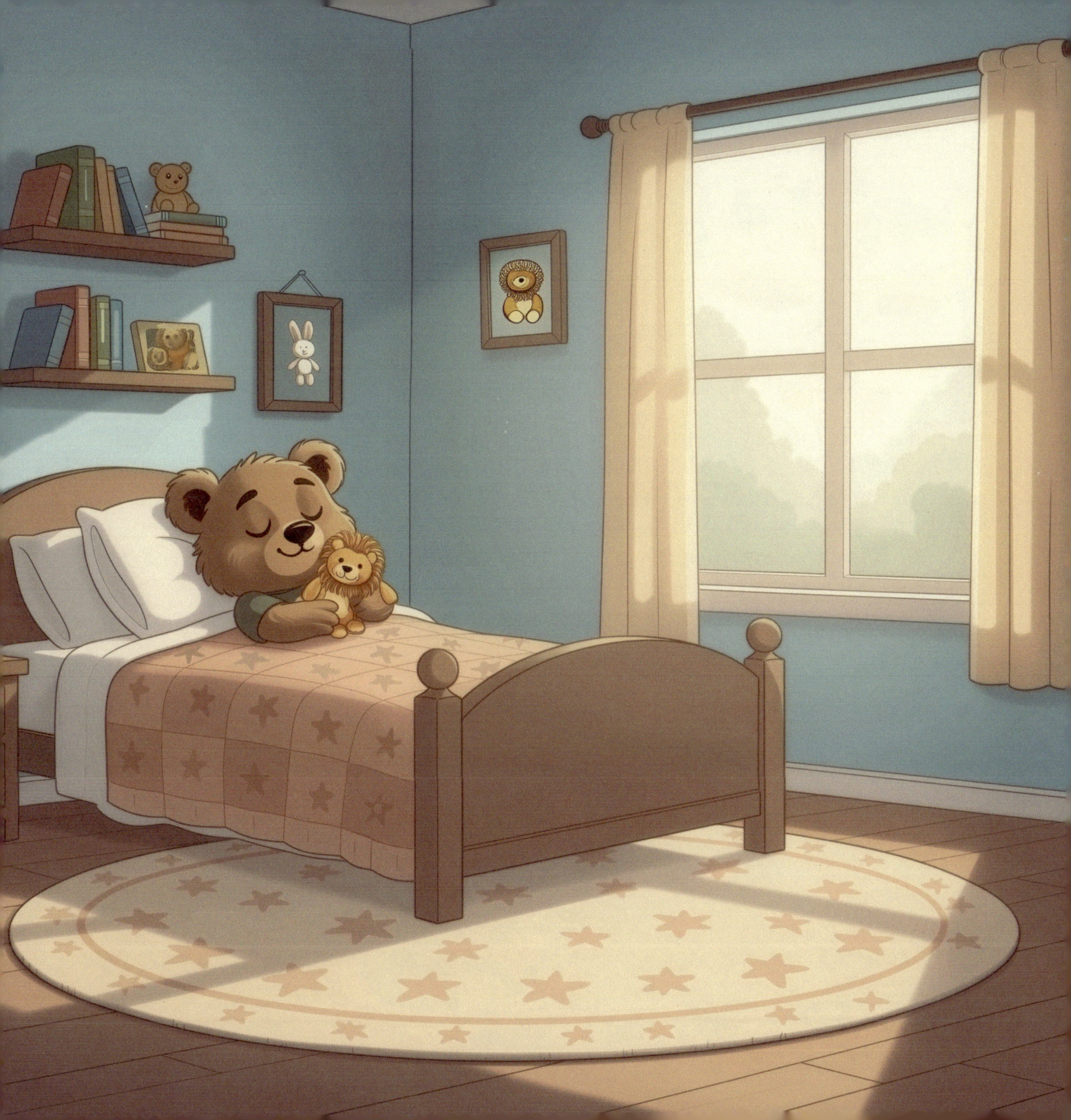

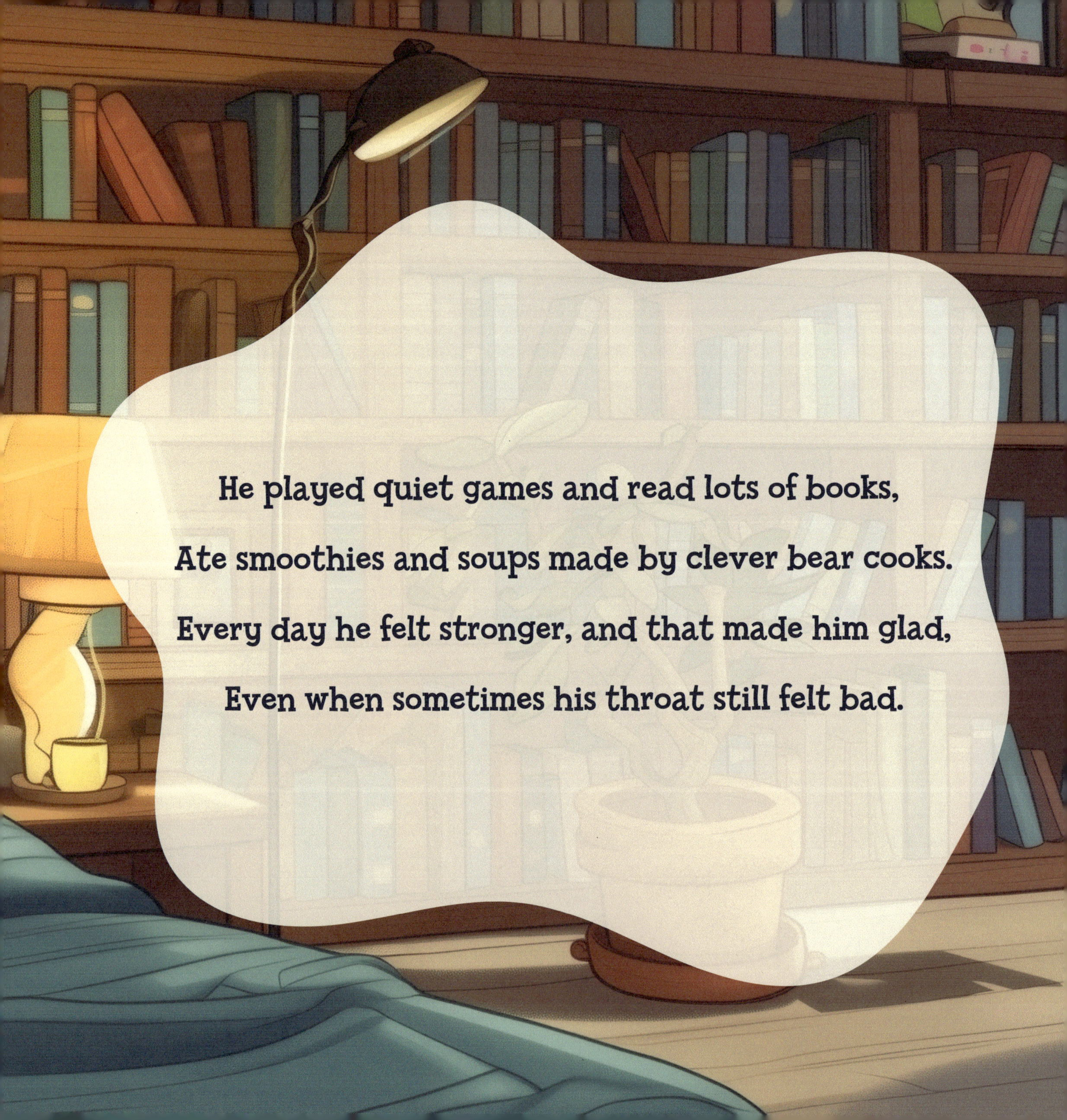

He played quiet games and read lots of books,
Ate smoothies and soups made by clever bear cooks.
Every day he felt stronger, and that made him glad,
Even when sometimes his throat still felt bad.

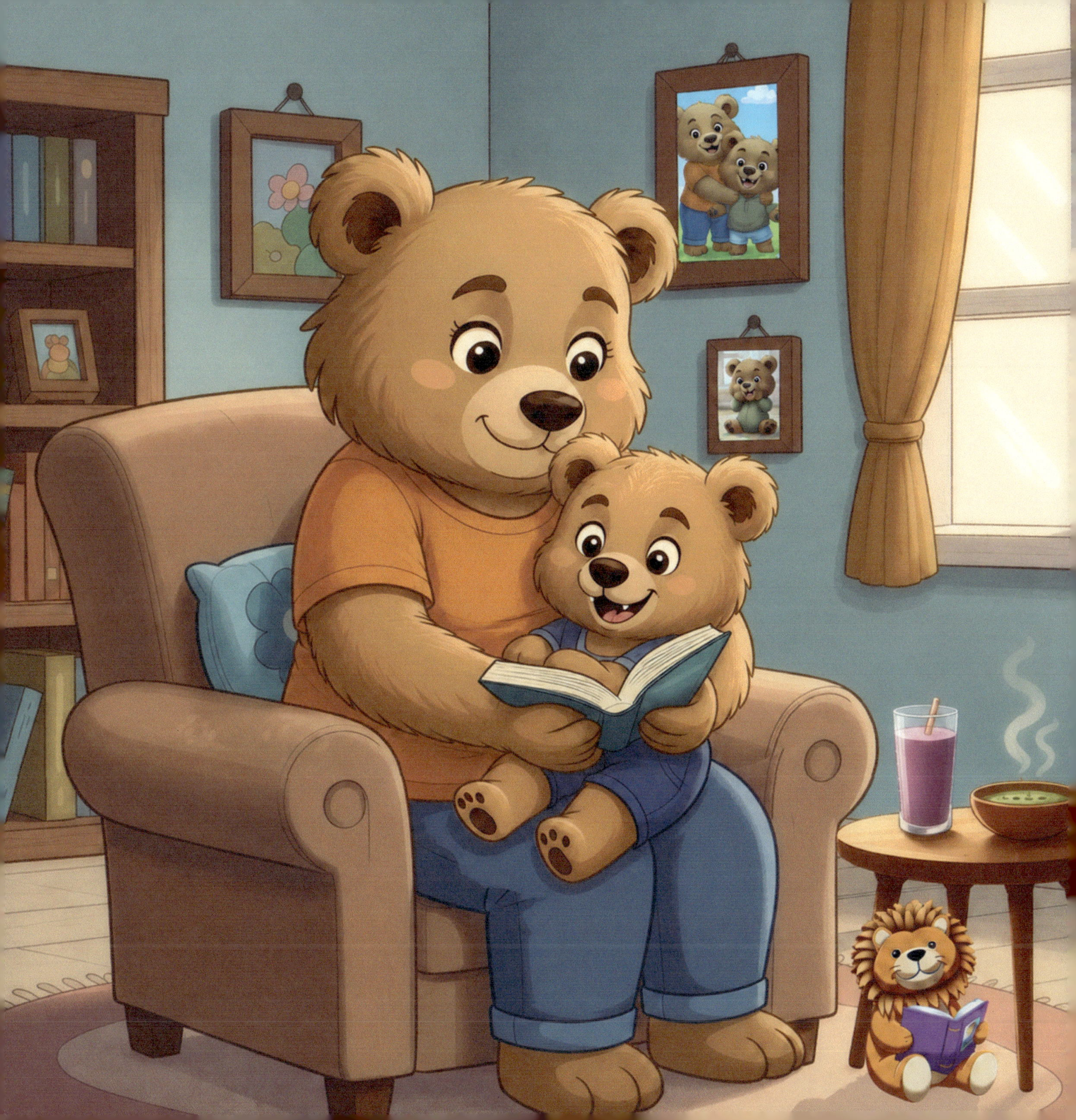

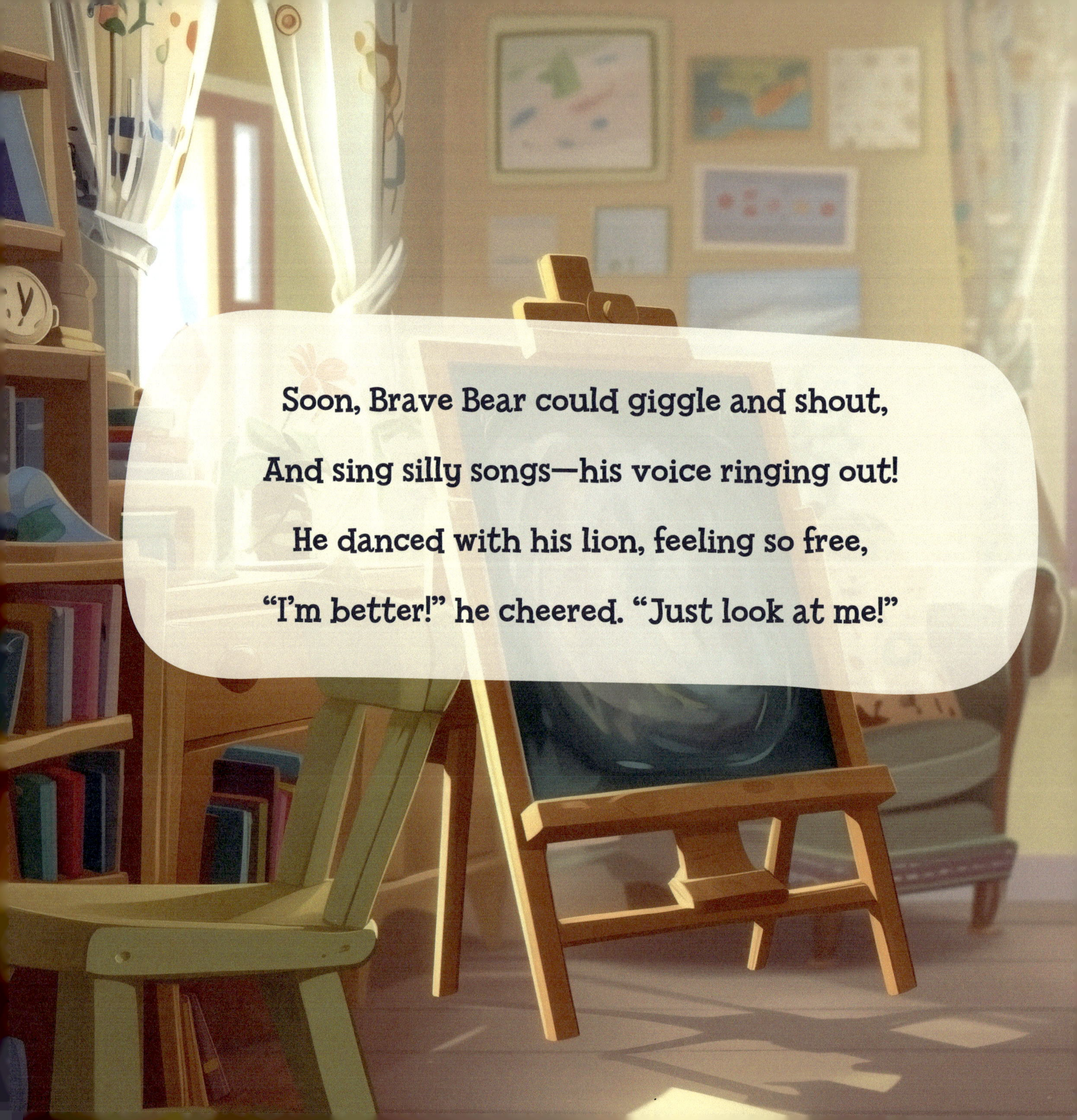

Soon, Brave Bear could giggle and shout,
And sing silly songs—his voice ringing out!
He danced with his lion, feeling so free,
"I'm better!" he cheered. "Just look at me!"

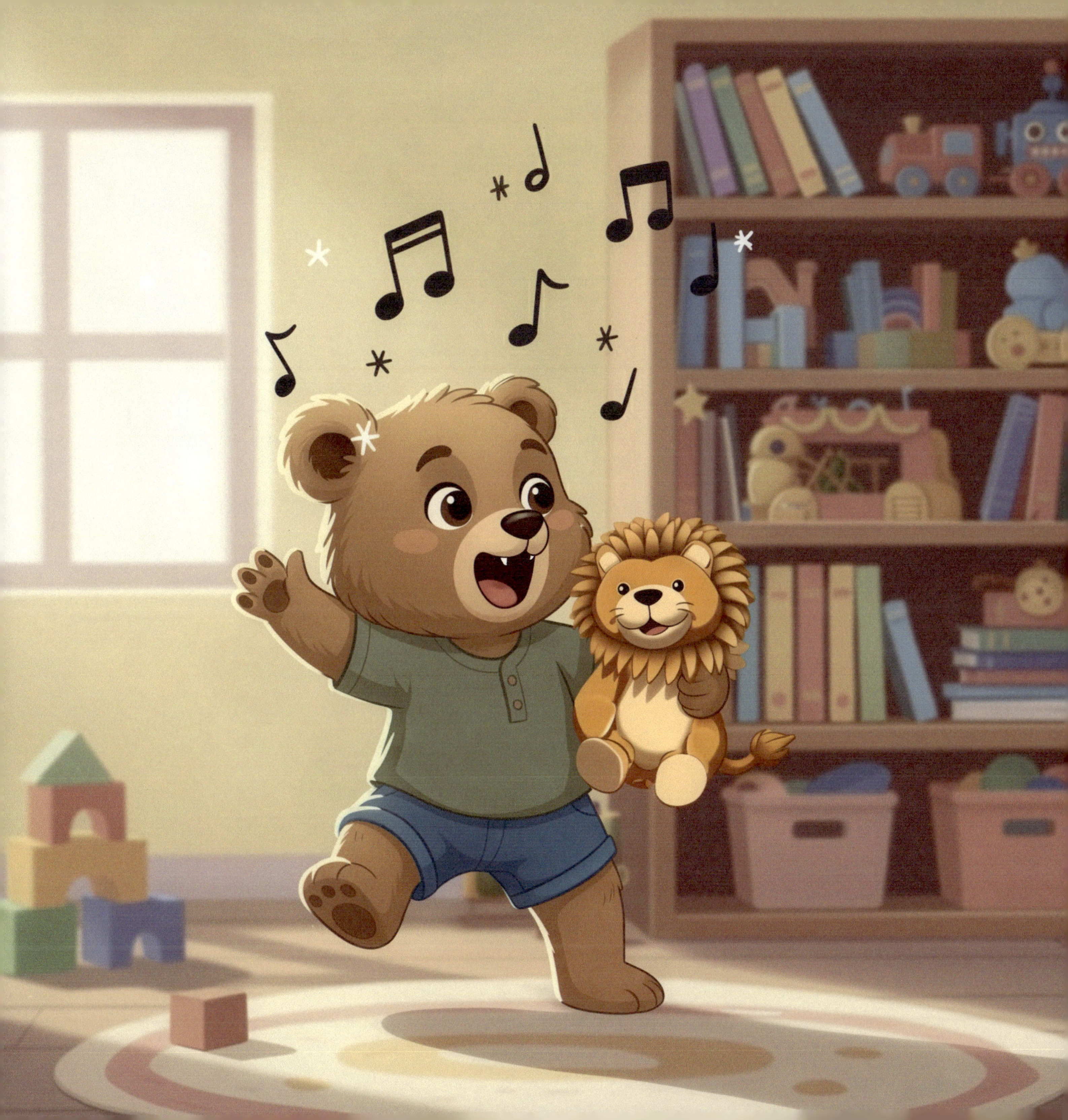

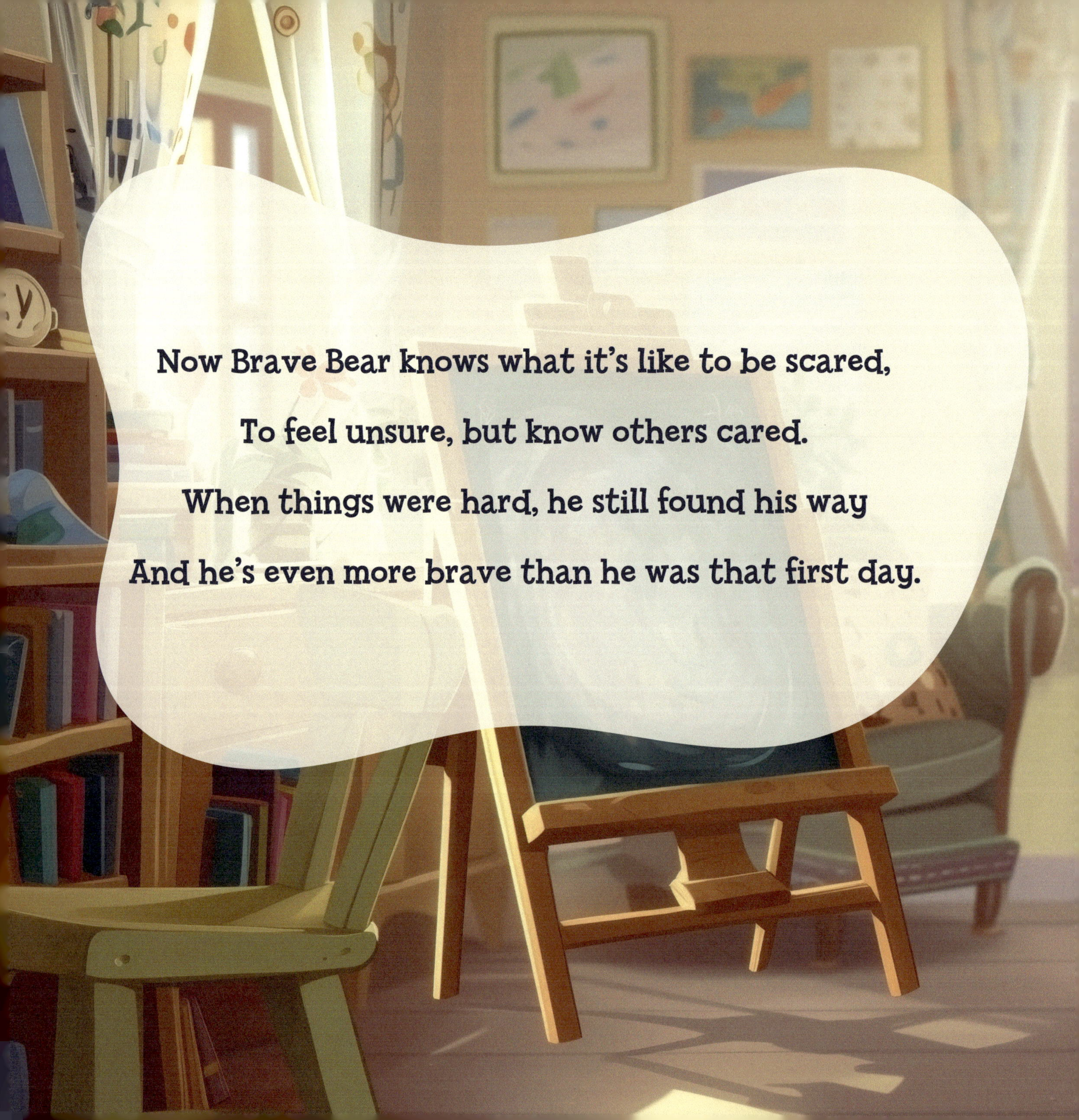

Now Brave Bear knows what it's like to be scared,

To feel unsure, but know others cared.

When things were hard, he still found his way

And he's even more brave than he was that first day.

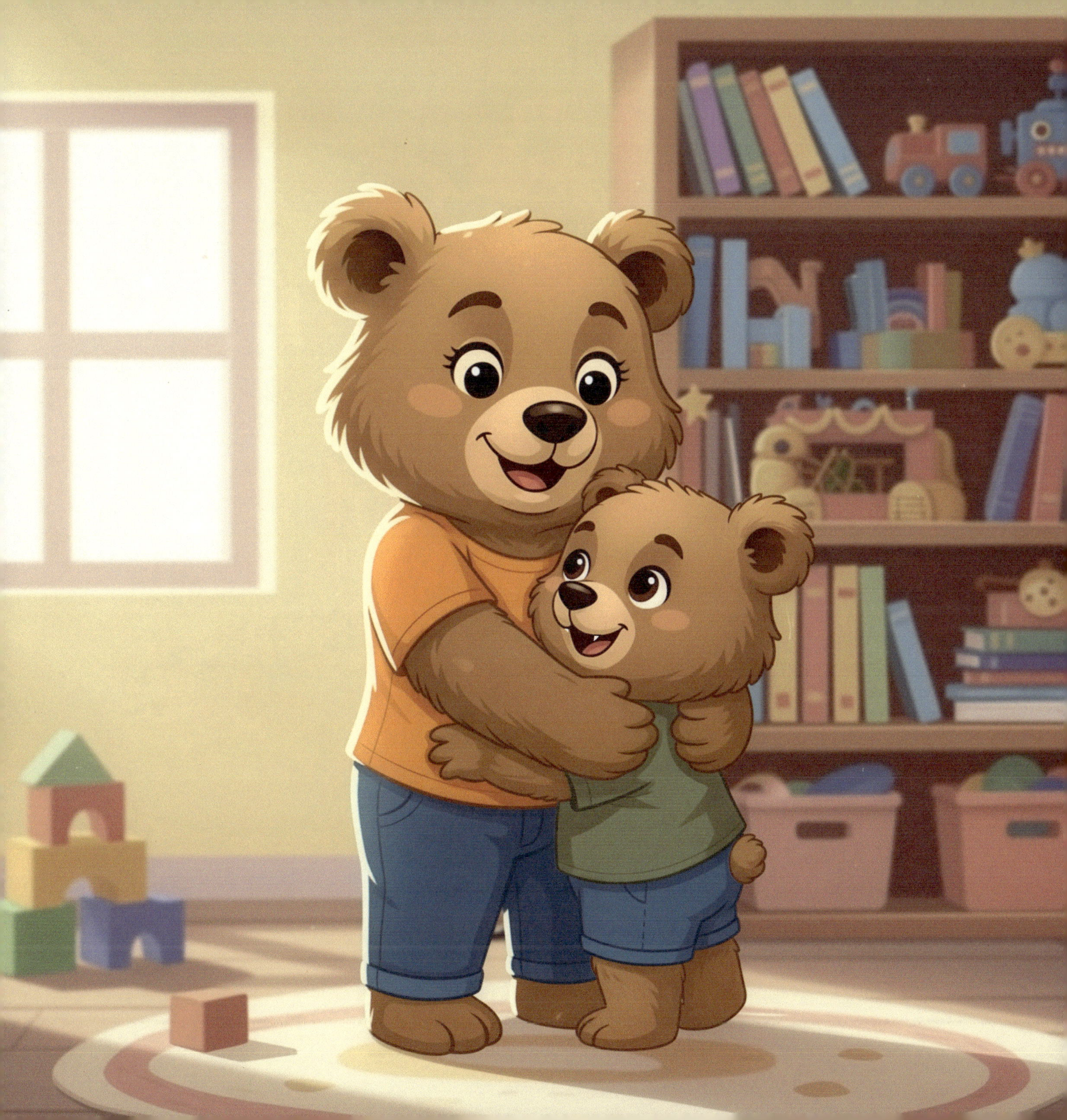

Brave Bear's Healing Tips

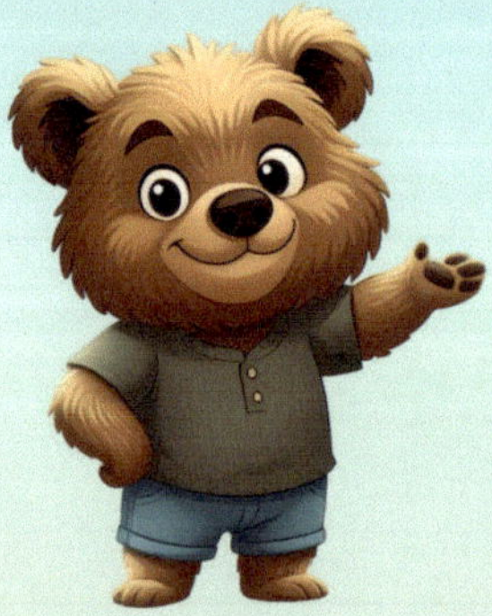

When bodies are healing,
they need extra care,
So here are some tips from
your friend, Brave Bear!

Listen to parents, they
know what to do.
They'll guide every step
and take care of you.

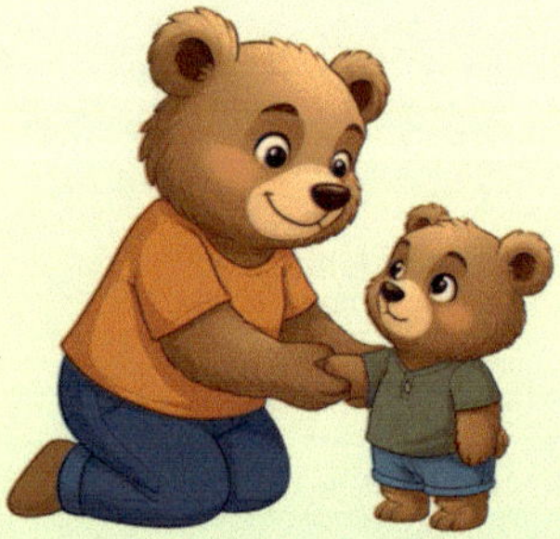

Drink water and juice,
take medicine too.
Both work together to
feel good as new.

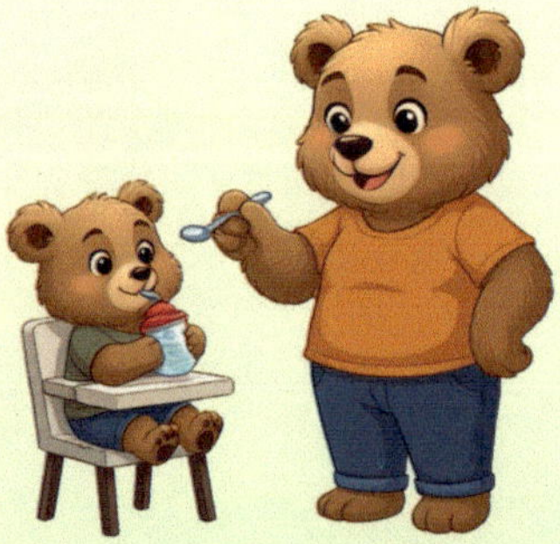

Rest when you're tired, let
dreams help you mend.
You're brave and you're
healing, my sweet
little friend.

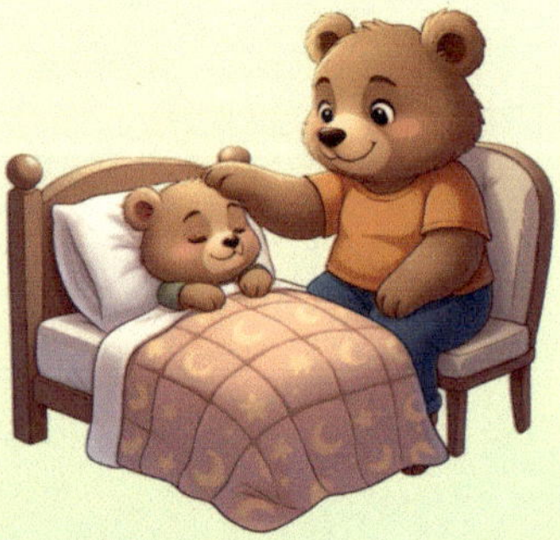

Certificate of Bravery

This certifies that

____

was so very brave during their tonsil surgery and recovery!

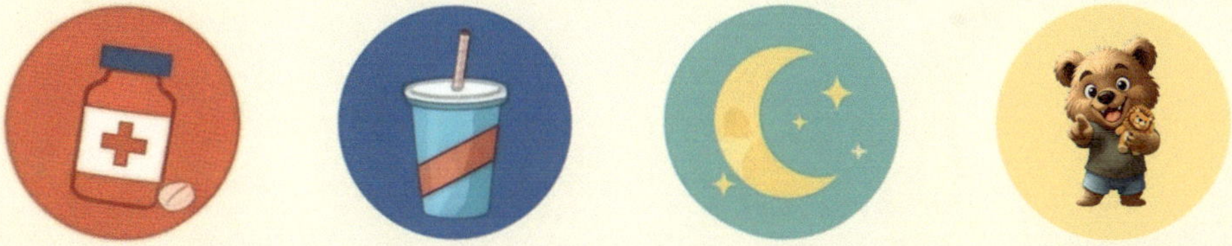

medicine water rest courage

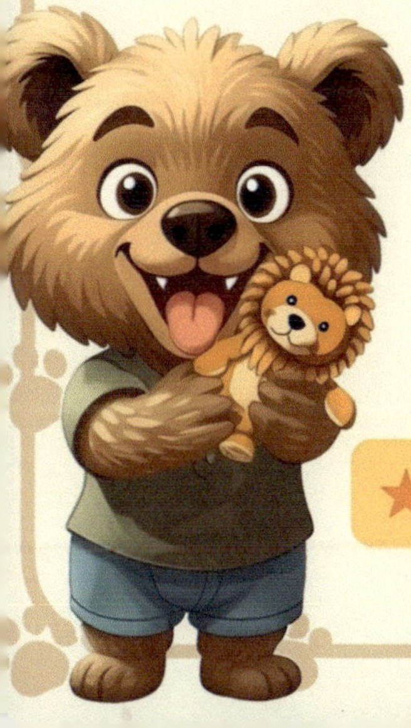

★ **You are a true Brave Little Patient!** ★

Date: ____________

Made in United States
Cleveland, OH
08 November 2026

47841301R00021